A CARBOHYDRATE COMPASS TO THE SUPERMARKET!

How simple! How basic! How essential! Finally, a carbohydrate gram counter that penetrates the mystery of brand-name foods. Finally, a complete counter that takes the monotony out of low-carbohydrate meals!

Aisle by aisle, shelf by shelf, THE BRAND-NAME CARBOHYDRATE GRAM COUNTER reveals all. Fresh foods, frozen foods, canned and convenience foods, snacks, specialties, delicacies, drinks—every gram count you want is here! Over 5500 listings; the best-known brands on the market; counts never published before!

"THE BRAND-NAME CARBOHYDRATE GRAM COUNTER fills a void. . . . Until now there has been a dearth of accurate information on the carbohydrate content of thousands of everyday foods. Those who find controlled-carbohydrate dieting more pleasant than controlled-calorie dieting will find Corinne Netzer's handbook convenient, comprehensive, and precise."

—From the preface by
Irwin M. Stillman, M.D.

THE BRAND-NAME CARBOHYDRATE GRAM COUNTER

By CORINNE T. NETZER

Preface by Irwin M. Stillman, M.D.

A DELL BOOK

Published by
Dell Publishing Co., Inc.
1 Dag Hammarskjold Plaza
New York, New York 10017

Printed in the United States of America

First printing—May 1973

For Alice Payton White

ACKNOWLEDGMENTS

A book of this scope isn't the result of just one person's efforts, or even one hundred people's efforts. An investigator of a field as broad as the commercial food industry must rely almost entirely on the goodwill and cooperation of the industry itself. Without that assistance, it would be impossible to compile a book such as this; therefore, I want to acknowledge my indebtedness to every company that responded to what must have seemed endless requests for data, clarification, more data and more clarification.

In addition, I am indebted to Evonne Rae, Elaine Chaback, Carol Robinson, and Meg Raben for their help in organizing what was a mountain of "raw" material.

C.T.N.

PREFACE

Readers who are familiar with my work in the field of overweight and with my books (*The Doctor's Quick Weight Loss Diet* and *The Doctor's Quick Inches-Off Diet*) are well aware of my conviction that obesity is this nation's foremost health hazard. Over the last three decades we have become a society that overeats and underexercises, and as a result we are now faced with what must be considered an obesity problem of epidemic proportions.

If you doubt the severity of the problem, bear in mind that among the serious disorders affected adversely by overweight are hypertension (high blood pressure), diabetes, and, most important, atherosclerosis (coronary artery disease). Right now the annual death rate for men aged fifty to fifty-nine from atherosclerosis and degenerative heart disease is higher in the United States than anywhere else in the world. Worse still, it is estimated that at age thirty or older, 30 percent of American men and 40 percent of American women are twenty or more pounds overweight. What is the relationship between overweight and coronary artery disease? It can be summed up this simply: The prevalence of coronary artery disease among Americans is lowest in people whose weight is below normal; the prevalence of the disease is highest in people who are overweight *and* increases proportionately with each excess pound. Unfortunately, there is still much to be learned about the causes of most kinds of heart disease, but there is uniform medical agreement that those who are overweight are more likely to be struck by a serious heart disorder than those whose weight is normal or less than normal.

If the above facts haven't convinced you of the urgency of reaching your proper weight, *and* maintaining it, consider these statistics, the result of studies by major life insurance companies: If you are 10 percent overweight, your expected life span is about 10 percent shorter; if you are 20 percent overweight, your expected life span is about 20 percent shorter, etc. For example, if you are a white American woman aged forty, your life expectancy is, according to the National Center for Health Statistics, 78.3 years; however, if you are 15 percent overweight, you are more likely to die at about age sixty-seven—a full eleven years before your time. If you are more than 15 percent overweight, your chance of dying prematurely increases proportionately.

These are grim statistics, but you should be aware of them. Wanting to look better is an excellent reason for dieting; wanting to live longer is an even better reason.

In my fifty years of medical practice, I have treated more than 10,000 overweight men and women, and, as a result, I am convinced of the success of fast-action dieting —particularly for those who have failed to reduce on lengthy regimens. Since the publication of my books, I have had an opportunity to speak to literally millions who are overweight; and no matter if I am on television or in a lecture hall or in a bookstore, I restate publicly what I have always told my patients privately: *Take that fat off fast; take it off on whatever diet suits you best.*

I recommend that you check with your own physician before starting on a specific diet, and I also recommend that you see him or her at reasonable intervals thereafter. In the vast majority of cases, your doctor will agree that the diet you've chosen is far healthier for you than continuing to overeat as you have.

In 1969, I consented to write a preface to Corinne Netzer's book, *The Brand-Name Calorie Counter*, because I felt it contained data that everyone, professionals in the field of health as well as the general public, could benefit from. My opinion of Mrs. Netzer's work was shared by many, among them Dr. Morris Fishbein, former editor of *JAMA* (*The Journal of the American Medical Association*) and present editor of *Medical World News*. In June 1969, Dr. Fishbein wrote in the latter publication: "For doctors trying to help patients manage a controlled-calorie diet regimen, help has appeared in a book that takes note of supermarket realities. . . . Now the overweight patient can count the calories in almost all prepared or convenience foods—and compare scores of various brands as well."

I've consented to write a preface to *The Brand-Name Carbohydrate Gram Counter* because I feel that this book too fills a void. In recent years there has been a surge of renewed interest in diets that are low in carbohydrate and high in protein and fat, but until now there has been a dearth of accurate information on the carbohydrate content of thousands of everyday foods. Those who find controlled-carbohydrate dieting more pleasant than controlled-calorie dieting will find this handbook convenient, comprehensive, and precise.

By the way, despite what you may have heard or read to the contrary, low-carbohydrate diets are neither new nor revolutionary. Indeed, the first widely known such diet dates back over one hundred years when a London physician, William Harvey, fashioned a low-carbohydrate regimen for a wealthy coffin-maker named William Banting. The Harvey diet added up to nearly 2,800 calories a day, and the obese Mr. Banting—who had failed to reduce on low-calorie plans—lost fifty pounds in a year. From that time until the present, variations of high-protein, low-carbohydrate diets have flourished. In 1967, I included four variations of these plans in *The Doctor's Quick Weight Loss Diet*, and I will be writing more on the subject in the near future.

For now, it is enough to say simply that if low-carbohydrate dieting works for you, and if your physician approves, stick with it. Remember, what matters most is to *get that fat off fast*—on whatever diet suits you best.

IRWIN M. STILLMAN, M.D.

INTRODUCTION

As you doubtless know already, low-carbohydrate dieting has little in common with low-calorie dieting. On a low-carb plan, you're allowed pure proteins (meat, fish, and poultry) to your stomach's content, plus goodies high in fat such as butter, heavy cream, Hollandaise, mayonnaise, and other foods usually forbidden on a diet. You lose weight by curtailing your intake of starches and sugars; you ignore calories; you count carbohydrate grams.

However, while low-carb reducing is unique in many ways, it is similar to low-calorie reducing in one unhappy respect: after a week or two, diet menus tend to be dismally, depressingly alike. Man (and woman) cannot live by steak alone, and in all too short a time the low-carb dieter is apt to grow faint at the sight of a Fig Newton or a Twinkie.

Take my word, I know. In 1970, I tried *Cosmopolitan*'s low-carb Ten-Day-Ten-Pounds-Off Diet, and while I lost weight on schedule (and was never actually hungry), I was maddened by a lust for Cracker Jacks. I owned a small carbohydrate gram counter, but it didn't list Cracker Jacks—or Vita herring in sour cream, or Kraft onion Ready Dip, or literally thousands of common, brand-name foods dear to the heart of any red-blooded American.

However, ten days is only one week, plus two days, plus 24 hours; I survived, *sans* Cracker Jacks, herring, onion Ready Dip, et al.

By the spring of 1971, I had, of course, regained the weight I'd lost in 1970 (the same ten pounds I'd lost the spring before and put back on during the winter of '69). It was diet time again. My choice for '71 was the highly acclaimed *Vogue* Super Diet—developed for *Vogue* by Dr. Robert C. Atkins, and later expanded into the best-selling book, *Dr. Atkins' Diet Revolution.* The *Vogue* 16-day low-carb plan worked even faster than promised, but again I was bedeviled by savage cravings, this time for Chipper crackers and Mallomars. Again, my little gram counter failed me; no listing for Mallomars; no Chipper crackers. And so the compilation of this book began.

Depending on the specific low-carb regimen you're following and/or how long you've been on it, there comes a time when you are allowed to "spend" some carbohydrate grams as you please. If you're on the Drinking Man's Diet, your allowance may be as high as 50 to 60 grams a day; if you're following Dr. Atkins' maintenance plan, your allowance may be 20 to 40 grams a day; but whatever the magic number, you need specific information to get the most from each of your precious grams.

This book contains that kind of information. It lists the number of carbohydrate grams in over 5500 foods and beverages, the vast majority of them familiar, brand-name products. What's more, it reveals the difference in carbohydrates that often exists between two or more brands or varieties of the "same" food. For example, consider something as seemingly simple as a cup of chicken noodle soup, either canned or made from a mix. How many grams of carbohydrate are there in a cup (eight fluid ounces) of prepared chicken noodle soup?

The *accurate* answer is anywhere from 4.4 grams (Manischewitz) to 5.0 grams (Wyler's) to 7.9 grams (Heinz

Chicken and Star Noodles) to 8.4 grams (Campbell's) to 8.8 grams (Golden Grain) to 8.9 grams (Lipton's) to 9.3 grams (Campbell's Noodle-O's) to 9.5 grams (Heinz). In short, the only way to determine—for sure—the number of carbohydrate grams in commercial chicken noodle soup is to know who made the soup.

Why is there such a surprising difference in the carbohydrate content of the "same" kinds of brand-name foods? For exactly the same reason that your homemade chicken salad, for example, is likely to contain fewer or more grams of carbohydrate than my homemade chicken salad: the recipes are different. Chances are, we begin with the same basics: chicken, hard-cooked eggs and mayonnaise, but if your recipe calls for green olives and diced celery and mine calls for chopped walnuts and sweet pickles, the finished foods are hardly the same. We've both made what is rightly called "chicken salad," but the taste *and* carbohydrate content of our two salads are appreciably different.

This same reasoning is applicable to the majority of brand-name foods we buy—particularly processed foods. Every company has its own recipe for each of its products; therefore, while there are many brands of the "same" foods, they are likely to vary in composition, taste, and carbohydrate gram content.

Just for the record, let me state clearly that I'm merely a dieter, not a dietician or nutritionist, and the aim of this book isn't to suggest to you how to reduce or what to eat. The kind of diet you undertake is a matter for you to decide for yourself—or, if there's any question about your health, with the aid of a physician. The sole aim of *The Brand-Name Carbohydrate Gram Counter* is to take some of the mystery (and monotony) out of low-gram eating.

I hope you will find all of your favorite brands included in these pages; however, the limitations of time and space are bound to cause some disappointments. In general, I've tried to include those products that are best known and most widely distributed; specifically, you may find a favorite food missing because 1) the company is in the process of reformulating the recipe; 2) the company lacks the facilities and/or the budget to analyze the product's nutritive values; 3) the product is available only locally, or in a very few other states; 4) the product, though still in some stores, has been discontinued.

If you're truly unhappy that some of your favorite foods aren't listed, I urge you to write to the companies that make them. In recent years, the food industry has recognized—and is responsive to—the consumer's right to information regarding the things we eat. Indeed, the Grocery Manufacturers of America, a trade association representing every major food producer in the United States, has stated publicly that "manufacturers are anxious to let you know about the contents and nutritive values of their products."

One group of foods you won't find listed in this book is diet products—No-Cal, for example. Nutritive values are stated clearly on every diet-food label I've ever seen; therefore, in order to include as many "regular" foods as possible, I've deliberately omitted all diet products.

As you will see, there are many ways to utilize the data made available here. For example, you may decide to try new foods and/or new brands; you may decide to succumb —or not to succumb—to an Aunt Jemima cinnamon stick (21 grams) or a Jeno's pepperoni pizza roll (3.8 grams). But whatever you decide, your choices will be based on an expanded—and accurate—knowledge of specific foods and their carbohydrate content.

C.T.N.

CONTENTS

HOW TO USE THIS BOOK

WHERE TO FIND WHAT

Most carbohydrate gram counters list foods alphabetically. This counter does not. It lists foods categorically. All cereals are grouped together; so are all lunch meats, all fruits, all vegetables, all wines, and so on. For example—and, more important, for convenience—if you want to find the gram content of various kinds of soups, you don't have to hopscotch from *A* (alphabet) through *W* (won ton); you simply turn to the chapter titled "Soups, Broths and Chowders," and there in one place you will find 210 soup listings—from alphabet through won ton.

Occasionally you may have trouble deciding what category a food belongs in; occasionally, too, the same food, in different forms, appears in more than one category. To locate hard-to-categorize and multiple-listed foods quickly, just flip to the index.

BE CAREFUL ABOUT MAKING COMPARISONS

It is only natural that you will want to use this counter to compare the carbohydrate content of different foods and different brands. In many instances, you can make comparisons accurately by merely glancing at the listings. For example, all soft drinks are listed in the same measure—eight fluid ounces; therefore, you can easily compare the gram content of Coca-Cola with that of Canada Dry Jamaican Cola, or Schweppes Bitter Lemon, or whatever.

To facilitate easy comparisons, categories have been listed in a uniform measure whenever it was possible or feasible to do so. However, it was neither feasible nor sensible to list certain foods in a uniform measure. For example, all data on crackers could have been presented in a measure of one ounce, but that would have meant you would have to weigh a Triscuit to learn its carbohydrate content. For practicality's sake, crackers, cookies, bread, and various other foods are listed by the piece—*in the size packaged by the manufacturer*. This means you can easily determine the number of grams in a single cracker, but you cannot compare different brands and varieties accurately. Why? Because, unless you weigh every cracker, you have no way of knowing if they are the same size.

To get the most from this book—and your diet—you must recognize that similar foods aren't necessarily packaged in the same or even similar sizes. For example, consider Pepperidge Farm's Party Pan finger roll and the same company's Party Pan round roll. A finger roll has 9.2 carbohydrate grams; a round roll has 5.5 carbohydrate grams—yet both rolls contain 14 carbohydrate grams per ounce. The answer to this seeming mystery is obvious: The finger roll is nearly twice the size of the round roll; therefore, its gram content is proportionately higher.

The point here is simple, but important. If you're not certain that products are the same size, *don't make comparisons; they may not be accurate.*

ANOTHER CAUTION ABOUT COMPARISONS

Because even doctors and home economists sometimes confuse measures by capacity with measures by weight, it should be noted also that you can't, for example, accu-

rately compare four ounces of spaghetti with half a cup
of boiled rice. Four ounces is a measure of how much
something weighs. Half a cup is a measure of how much
space something occupies. The units of measure are dis-
similar and, therefore, not comparable. Think of it this
way: Eight ounces of plain popped popcorn contains 174
grams of carbohydrates and fills the capacity of nearly 17
eight-ounce measuring cups; an eight-ounce cupful of plain
popped popcorn contains 10.3 grams of carbohydrates and
weighs less than half an ounce. Clearly, eight ounces of
popcorn and an eight-ounce cupful of popcorn are not the
same!

Sometimes exactly eight ounces of a food exactly fills
the capacity of an eight-ounce cup, but more often it does
not—which is why you shouldn't try to compare foods
listed by weight with foods listed by volume. Just remember: The capacity of a standard eight-ounce measuring
cup is eight *fluid* ounces, not eight weight ounces.

You can, of course, compare the gram content of foods
listed in the same unit of measure—and you can, of course,
convert a unit of measure to a smaller or larger amount.
The charts below will help to make such conversions.

EQUIVALENTS BY CAPACITY
(all measurements level)

1 quart = 32 fluid ounces
= 4 cups
1 cup = 8 fluid ounces
= ½ pint
= 16 tablespoons
1 tablespoon = 3 teaspoons

EQUIVALENTS BY WEIGHT

1 pound = 16 ounces
3.52 ounces = 100 grams*
1 ounce = 28.35 grams*

* *Metric weight grams; not carbohydrate grams.*

PAY ATTENTION TO PACKAGE SIZES

To get full value from *The Brand-Name Carbohydrate Gram Counter*, it's important that you pay attention to package sizes. Specifically, whenever the gram content of a food is listed by one ounce, you must check the food's label to learn how much the product weighs—and then multiply its weight in ounces by the number of carbohydrate grams per ounce. Cheeses, for example, are listed in a one-ounce measure. To determine the carbohydrate content of an eight-ounce package of Kraft processed American cheese, simply multiply eight by .5, and you will see that the entire package contains only four grams of carbohydrate.

Pay attention to weights too whenever a product is listed by the whole package. For example, as this book goes to press, the weight of Banquet's Cookin' Bag meat loaf entree is five ounces—and the data herein pertains to the full five ounces. Should Banquet increase or decrease the amount of meat loaf in Cookin' Bags, the data should be adjusted accordingly.

PAY ATTENTION TO PACKAGE DIRECTIONS

You will find many products listed in this counter that require some home preparation: condensed soups, salad dressing mixes, so-called "dinner" mixes, and more. For convenience, the data on the majority of these products is given for the "finished" food when it is prepared *according to package directions*. Should you make a change in a package recipe, bear in mind that you may also charge the carbohydrate content of the finished food. For example, if a package recipe calls for a cup of whole milk and you substitute a cup of heavy cream, the prepared food will have a lower carbohydrate content than is listed here. There is no reason why you shouldn't vary package directions; the point is, if you do, be sure to determine how the change affects the gram content of the prepared food.

SOURCES AND ACCURACY OF DATA

Carbohydrate values listed in this book are based on two sources: 1) data obtained from the producers and processors of all brand-name foods; 2) data obtained from United States Department of Agriculture publications pertaining to the nutritive composition of basic and other foods. Every care has been exercised to evaluate the data as accurately and fully as possible; every effort has been made to present the material clearly and usefully.

Consumers should be aware, however, that a variety of factors can, to some extent, affect the accuracy of any and all analyses of food. For example, apples grown in different regions of the country may differ slightly in composition; therefore, the carbohydrate value shown for apples, or for any product that contains apples, must be considered average or typical. Seasonal changes can also affect the composition of an apple; so too can the maturity of the crop when picked. For these and similar reasons, and because there is no practical way to analyze every sample of a pure or processed food, it is an accepted practice within the food industry—and within the U.S. Department of Agriculture—to present nutritive data that is typical or "proximate."

As this unabridged edition of *The Brand-Name Carbohydrate Gram Counter* goes to press, the data has been checked (and, where necessary, revised) to see that it is as up-to-date as possible. However, just as you strive to vary or improve your recipes, so do home economists in the food industry; therefore, it's impossible to guarantee that some of the data won't change in time. As needed, corrections will be made in later editions of the book. Until then, you must be on the lookout for changes yourself. In particular, if you find that a favorite food is suddenly labeled "New" or "Improved," you may want to write the producer to ask if the food's carbohydrate content has changed.

ABBREVIATIONS
USED IN THIS BOOK

cond. . . . . condensed
e.g. . . . . for example
fl. . . . . fluid
" . . . . inch
lb. . . . . pound
oz. . . . . ounce
pkg. . . . . package
swt. . . . . sweetened
unswt. . . . . unsweetened
tr. . . . . trace*
tbsp. . . . . tablespoon
tsp. . . . . teaspoon
w/ . . . . with
wo/ . . . . without

Less than one-tenth (.1) of one gram

CHAPTER 1

FRUITS
AND FRUIT PRODUCTS

FRUITS, FRESH*, half cup, except as noted

See also "Fruits, Canned, Dried & Frozen"

	GRAMS
apples, w/skin, 1 medium (about 3 per lb.)	20.0
applies, wo/skin, 1 medium (about 3 per lb.)	18.3
apples, pared, diced	7.7
apricots, 1 average (about 12 per lb.)	4.6
avocados, California, cubed	4.6
avocados, Florida, cubed	6.7
bananas, 1 medium (about 3 per lb.)	22.6
bananas, sliced	16.7
bananas, plantain, 1 medium (about 3 per lb.)	33.7
blackberries	9.2
blueberries	10.9
cantaloupe, ¼ melon, 5″ diameter	7.2
cantaloupe, balls or cubes	6.2
cherries, sour	8.5
cherries, sweet	10.2
coconut, ¼ lb. meat	21.0
coconut, shredded	3.9
crab apples, ¼ lb.	18.5
currants, red or white	6.6

Fruits, Fresh, continued

figs, 1 small (about 12 per lb.) 7.7
gooseberries 7.2
grapefruit:
   pink, ½ medium, 4½" diameter 15.1
   white, seeded, ½ medium, 4½" diameter 13.8
   white, seedless, ½ medium, 4½" diameter 12.6
   white sections 9.8
grapes, American types (Concord, Delaware, Niagara, etc.) 7.5
grapes, European types (Malaga, Muscat, Thompson, Tokay, etc.) ..12.3
guavas, 1 small 11.7
honeydew, ¼ wedge of 1-lb. melon 5.5
lemons, 1 medium, 2" diameter 5.0
limes, 1 large, 2" diameter 5.6
loganberries 10.7
mangoes, 1 medium, 3¾" long 34.1
nectarines, 1 medium (about 5 per lb.) 14.3
oranges, California Navel, 1 medium, 2-4/5" diameter 16.0
oranges, Florida, all varieties, 1 medium, 3" diameter 19.0
orange sections, California Navel 15.5
orange sections, California Valencia 15.1
orange sections, Florida varieties 14.6
papayas, cubed 9.1
peaches, 1 medium (about 4 per lb.) 10.0
peaches, sliced 8.2
pears, 1 large (about 2 per lb.) 31.6
persimmons, Japanese or Kaki, 1 medium, 2½" diameter 20.0
pineapple, diced 9.6
plums, Damson, 1 average (about 7 per lb.) 10.5
raspberries, black 9.7
raspberries, red 8.4
rhubarb, cubed 2.1
strawberries, whole 6.3
tangerines, 1 average (about 4 per lb.) 9.7
watermelon, balls or cubes 5.1

* *Data from United States Department of Agriculture*

FRUITS, CANNED, DRIED & FROZEN, half cup, except as noted

See also "Fruits, Fresh"

	GRAMS
apples, dried, uncooked (Del Monte)	27.3
apples, dried, cooked, unswt.*	26.3
apples, dried, cooked, swt.*	40.8
apple fritters, frozen (Mrs. Paul's), 12-oz. pkg.	96.6
apple rings, spiced, w/syrup, canned (Musselman's), 4 rings**	20.8
apple slices, w/syrup, canned (Musselman's)	26.9
applesauce, sweetened, canned or in jars:	
(Del Monte)	32.5
(Hunt's Snack Pack), 5-oz. can	24.4
(Mott's)	26.2
(Mott's Country Style with Cinnamon)	26.2
(Mott's Golden Delicious)	26.2
(Mott's McIntosh)	26.2
(Musselman's)	26.9
(Stokely-Van Camp)	27.4
apple-apricot sauce, swt., in jars (Mott's Fruit Treats)	25.8
apple-cherry sauce, swt., in jars (Mott's Fruit Treats)	26.9
apple-pineapple sauce, swt., in jars (Mott's Fruit Treats)	31.2
apple-raspberry sauce, swt., in jars (Mott's Fruit Treats)	27.8
apple-strawberry sauce, swt., in jars (Mott's Fruit Treats)	25.8
apricots:	
dried, uncooked (Del Monte), 4 oz.	69.7
dried, uncooked (Sunsweet), 4 oz.	68.9
dried, cooked, unswt.*	30.8
dried, cooked, swt.*	44.6
w/juice, canned (Libby's)	27.0
w/syrup, canned (Del Monte)	27.5
w/syrup, canned (Hunt's)	26.4
w/syrup, canned (Stokely-Van Camp—whole or halves)	23.6
blackberries, w/syrup, canned (Musselman's)	23.6
blueberries, w/syrup, canned (Musselman's)	25.6
blueberries, w/syrup, frozen (Birds Eye Quick Thaw)	28.7

Fruits, Canned, Dried & Frozen, continued

blueberries, wo/syrup, frozen (Seabrook Farms) 11.0
cherries:
    maraschino, in jars (Puresun), 1 average cherry** 1.7
    sour, w/syrup, canned (Stokely-Van Camp) 12.8
    sweet, w/syrup, canned (Musselman's) 20.5
    sweet, dark, w/syrup, canned (Del Monte) 23.5
    sweet, dark, w/syrup, canned (Stokely-Van Camp) 19.9
    sweet, light, w/syrup, canned (Del Monte Royal Anne) 28.1
    sweet, light, w/syrup, canned (Stokely-Van Camp) 19.9
    sweet, w/syrup, frozen (Birds Eye Quick Thaw) 30.8
coconut, swt., see "Sweet Baking Ingredients," page 193
crab apples, w/syrup, canned (Musselman's), 1 apple** 8.7
cranberry sauce, whole berry, canned (Ocean Spray), 4 oz.† 44.4
cranberry sauce, jellied, canned (Ocean Spray), 4 oz.† 42.8
currants, dried (Del Monte Zante), 4 oz. 86.0
dates, dried:
    whole, pitted (Bordo) 57.1
    whole, pitted (Dromedary) 56.2
    chopped (Dromedary) 57.1
    diced (Bordo) 57.1
figs, dried, 4 oz.* 78.3
figs, w/syrup, canned (Del Monte) 27.4
fruit, mixed, dried (Del Monte) 59.5
fruit, mixed, w/syrup, frozen (Birds Eye Quick Thaw) 28.4
fruit cocktail:
    w/juice, canned (Libby's) 22.0
    w/syrup, canned (Del Monte) 23.5
    w/syrup, canned (Hunt's) 29.8
    w/syrup, canned (Stokely-Van Camp) 23.2
fruit cup, w/syrup, canned (Del Monte), 5-oz. can 27.4
fruit cup, w/syrup, canned (Hunt's Snack Pack), 5-oz. can 24.8
fruit salad, w/juice, fresh, in jars (Kraft) 11.1
fruit salad, tropical, w/syrup, canned (Del Monte) 29.3
fruits for salad, w/syrup, canned (Del Monte) 21.4
grapefruit sections:
    unswt., fresh, in jars (Kraft) 8.3

grapefruit sections, continued

swt., fresh, in jars (Kraft) 10.0
swt., w/juice, canned (Del Monte) 10.4
swt., w/syrup, canned (Del Monte) 18.5
swt., w/syrup, canned (Stokely-Van Camp) 14.4
grapes, w/syrup, canned, Thompson seedless* 20.0
oranges, Mandarin, w/syrup, canned (Del Monte) 20.6
peaches:
dried, uncooked (Del Monte), 4 oz. 65.7
dried, uncooked (Sunsweet), 4 oz. 71.4
dried, cooked, unswt.* 30.0
dried, cooked, swt.* 43.1
w/juice, canned (Libby's) 30.0
w/syrup, canned (Del Monte), 5¼-oz. can 29.5
w/syrup, canned (Del Monte Cling) 26.1
w/syrup, canned (Del Monte Freestone) 29.1
w/syrup, canned (Heart's Delight Elberta Freestone) 23.9
w/syrup, canned (Hunt's Cling) 25.2
w/syrup, canned (Hunt's Snack Pack), 5-oz. can 27.7
w/syrup, canned (Stokely-Van Camp Cling—halves or slices) ... 22.8
w/syrup, canned
(Stokely-Van Camp Freestone—halves or slices) 22.8
w/syrup, frozen (Birds Eye Quick Thaw) 22.3
w/syrup, frozen (Seabrook Farms) 28.0
spiced, w/syrup, canned (Del Monte) 29.5
pears:
dried, uncooked (Del Monte), 4 oz. 65.8
dried, uncooked (Sunsweet), 4 oz. 71.2
dried, cooked, unswt.* 41.2
dried, cooked, swt.* 53.2
w/juice, canned (Libby's) 20.5
w/syrup, canned (Del Monte) 21.7
w/syrup, canned (Hunt's) 23.3
w/syrup, canned (Stokely-Van Camp) 22.1
pineapple:
chunks, w/juice, canned (Del Monte) 20.7
chunks, w/juice, canned (Dole) 17.1

pineapple, continued

chunks, w/heavy syrup, canned (Del Monte) 26.7
chunks, w/heavy syrup, canned (Dole) 22.0
chunks, w/heavy syrup, canned (Stokely-Van Camp) 21.8
chunks, w/heavy syrup, frozen (Dole) 22.0
chunks, w/extra heavy syrup, canned (Dole) 26.5
crushed, w/juice, canned (Dole) 17.1
crushed, w/heavy syrup, canned (Dole) 22.0
crushed, w/extra heavy syrup, canned (Stokely-Van Camp) 26.0
sliced, w/juice, canned (Dole), 1 slice 8.6
sliced, w/heavy syrup, canned
    (Dole—#1, #1½ or #2 can size), 1 slice 11.3
sliced, w/heavy syrup, canned (Dole—#1¼ can size), 1 slice ..19.5
sliced, w/heavy syrup, canned (Dole—#2½ can size), 1 slice ..20.3
sliced, w/extra heavy syrup, canned
    (Stokely-Van Camp), 1 slice 11.7
tidbits, w/heavy syrup, canned (Dole) 22.0
plums, w/syrup, canned (Del Monte) 30.4
plums, w/syrup, canned (Musselman's) 25.5
plums, w/syrup, canned (Stokely-Van Camp) 23.4
prunes:
dried, uncooked (Del Monte), 4 oz. 71.2
dried, uncooked (Del Monte Moist-Pak), 4 oz. 70.2
dried, uncooked (Sunsweet), 4 oz. 71.3
stewed, w/syrup, canned (Del Monte) 41.8
stewed, w/syrup, canned (Heart's Delight) 35.0
pitted, stewed, w/syrup, canned (Del Monte) 37.5
raisins, seedless (Del Monte Golden), 4 oz. 87.8
raisins, seedless (Del Monte Thompson), 4 oz. 87.9
raisins, seedless (Sun Maid), 4 oz. 87.5
raspberries, black, w/syrup, canned (Musselman's) 24.1
raspberries, red, w/syrup, frozen (Birds Eye Quick Thaw) 37.2
raspberries, red, w/syrup, frozen (Seabrook Farms) 31.0
rhubarb, w/syrup, frozen (Birds Eye) 21.4
strawberries:
w/syrup, frozen (Birds Eye Quick Thaw) 30.7
w/syrup, frozen (Birds Eye—halves) 39.9

strawberries, continued

w/syrup, frozen (Seabrook Farms) 36.0

wo/syrup, frozen (Seabrook Farms—whole) 10.0

* *Data from United States Department of Agriculture*
** *Drained of syrup*
† *Scant half cup*

FRUIT JUICES, six-ounce glass, except as noted

See also "Fruit & Fruit-Flavored Drinks"
and "Vegetable Juices"

	GRAMS
apple, bottled or canned (Mott's)	21.9
apple, bottled or canned (Musselman's)	19.5
apple, dairy-pack (Sealtest), 4-oz. container	15.1
fig, bottled (RealFig)	30.0
fig and prune, bottled (Fig 'N Prune)	30.0
grape:	
bottled (Welch's)	32.0
frozen, reconstituted* (Minute Maid)	25.0
frozen, reconstituted* (Snow Crop)	25.0
frozen, reconstituted* (Welch's)	22.5
grapefruit:	
fresh-squeezed**	17.0
canned (Del Monte)	17.6
canned (Libby's)	15.3
canned (Stokely-Van Camp)	15.0
dairy-pack (Kraft)	16.6
dairy-pack (Sealtest), 4-oz. container	12.0
dairy-pack (Tropicana)	19.0
frozen, reconstituted* (Minute Maid)	18.3
frozen, reconstituted* (Snow Crop)	18.3
swt., canned (Del Monte)	19.1
swt., canned (Stokely-Van Camp)	19.2

grapefruit, continued

swt., dairy-pack (Kraft)	20.8
swt., frozen, reconstituted* (Minute Maid)	22.3
swt., frozen, reconstituted* (Snow Crop)	22.3

lemon:

fresh-squeezed**, 2 tbsp.	2.4
bottled (ReaLemon), 2 tbsp.	2.0
bottled (Rose's), 2 tbsp.	2.6
frozen, reconstituted* (Minute Maid), 2 tbsp.	1.1
frozen, reconstituted* (Snow Crop), 2 tbsp.	1.1
lime, fresh-squeezed**, 2 tbsp.	2.7
lime, bottled (ReaLime), 2 tbsp.	3.0
lime, swt., bottled (Rose's), 2 tbsp.	12.0

orange:

fresh-squeezed, California Navel**	21.0
fresh-squeezed, California Valencia**	19.5
fresh-squeezed, Florida, most varieties, except Temple**	18.6
fresh-squeezed, Florida Temple**	24.0
canned (Del Monte)	23.5
canned (Libby's)	19.0
dairy-pack (Foremost)	23.9
dairy-pack (Kraft—fresh)	20.6
dairy-pack (Kraft—from concentrate)	22.2
dairy-pack (Pet)	17.8
dairy-pack (Sealtest)	21.7
dairy-pack (Sealtest), 4-oz. container	13.3
dairy-pack (Tropicana)	20.0
frozen, reconstituted* (Birds Eye)	20.0
frozen, reconstituted* (Libby's)	19.0
frozen, reconstituted* (Minute Maid)	21.4
frozen, reconstituted* (Snow Crop)	21.4
frozen, reconstituted* (Stokely-Van Camp)	22.0
swt., canned (Del Monte)	29.9
imitation, frozen, reconstituted* (Awake)	18.9
imitation, frozen, reconstituted* (Orange Plus)	24.9

orange-grapefruit:

canned (Stokely-Van Camp Citrusip)	16.6

orange-grapefruit juice, continued

    dairy-pack (Kraft) 21.1
    frozen, reconstituted* (Minute Maid) 19.1
    frozen, reconstituted* (Snow Crop) 19.1
    swt., canned (Stokely-Van Camp Citrusip) 19.2
orange-pineapple, dairy-pack (Kraft) 22.4
pineapple:
    canned (Del Monte) 24.3
    canned (Dole) 23.0
    canned (Stokely-Van Camp) 26.6
    frozen, reconstituted* (Dole) 23.3
pineapple-grapefruit, frozen, reconstituted* (Dole) 21.6
pineapple-orange, frozen, reconstituted* (Dole) 21.6
prune:
    bottled (RealPrune) 33.0
    bottled or canned (Sunsweet) 28.4
    canned (Del Monte) 23.3
    canned (Lady Betty) 31.0
    dairy-pack (Sealtest), 4-oz. container 23.0
    w/lemon, bottled or canned (Sunsweet) 28.4
    apricot-apple, bottled (Sunsweet) 24.0
tangerine, frozen, reconstituted* (Minute Maid) 20.8
tangerine, frozen, reconstituted* (Snow Crop) 20.8

  * *According to package directions*
  ** *Data from United States Department of Agriculture*

FRUIT & FRUIT-FLAVORED DRINKS, eight-ounce glass

See also "Fruit Juices" and "Soft Drinks & Mixers"

	GRAMS
apple, canned (Del Monte)	31.4
apple, canned (Hi-C)	29.7
apple-cranberry, bottled or canned (Mott's)	31.7
apple-grape, bottled or canned (Welch's)	32.0

Fruit & Fruit-Flavored Drinks, continued

apricot nectar, canned (Del Monte) 35.9
apricot nectar, canned (Heart's Delight) 36.3
apricot nectar, canned (Sunsweet) 36.0
apricot-apple, canned (BC) 32.6
berry, wild, canned (Hi-C) 30.3
cherry, canned (Hi-C) 30.3
cherry flavor, canned (Hi-C) 30.3
cherry flavor, mix, prepared* (Kool-Aid—regular) 25.0
cherry flavor, mix, prepared* (Kool-Aid—sugar swt.) 23.0
cherry-apple, canned (BC) 35.0
cherry, black, mix, prepared* (Kool-Aid) 25.0
cider, sweet, bottled (Mott's) 29.2
cider, cherry flavor, bottled (Mott's) 29.2
cider, cranberry flavor, bottled (Mott's) 29.2
citrus, canned (Hi-C Cooler) 30.3
cranberry cocktail, bottled (Ocean Spray) 38.0
cranberry-apple, bottled (Cranapple) 46.0
cranberry-grape, bottled (Grapeberry) 39.1
cranberry-orange flavor, mix, prepared* (Knox Gelatin) 28.0
cranberry-prune, bottled (Cranprune) 40.1
grape:
   canned (Del Monte) 32.8
   canned (Hi-C) 29.0
   canned (Stokely-Van Camp) 28.7
   dairy-pack (Tropicana) 26.6
   frozen, reconstituted* (Welch's) 30.0
grape flavor:
   mix, prepared* (Knox Gelatin) 23.4
   mix, prepared* (Kool-Aid—regular) 25.0
   mix, prepared* (Kool-Aid—sugar swt.) 23.0
   mix, prepared* (Salada) 24.7
   mix, prepared* (Tang) 31.6
   mix, prepared* (Wyler's) 21.0
grapeade, canned (Welchade) 31.0
grapeade, dairy-pack (Sealtest) 32.4
grapeade, w/lemon, frozen, reconstituted* (Welchade) 30.0

Fruit & Fruit-Flavored Drinks, continued

grape-apple, canned (BC) 36.9

grapefruit, dairy-pack (Tropicana) 26.6

grapefruit flavor, mix, prepared* (Tang) 30.0

lemon, dairy-pack (Sealtest) 30.1

lemonade:

    bottled or canned (Stokely-Van Camp) 28.0

    dairy-pack (Borden) 26.7

    dairy-pack (Sealtest) 26.7

    frozen, reconstituted* (Libby's) 22.1

    frozen, reconstituted* (Minute Maid) 26.1

    frozen, reconstituted* (ReaLemon) 32.0

    frozen, reconstituted* (Snow Crop) 26.1

    imitation, mix, prepared* (Kool-Aid—regular) 25.0

    imitation, mix, prepared* (Kool-Aid—sugar swt.) 23.0

    imitation, mix, prepared* (Salada) 23.9

    imitation, mix, prepared* (Wyler's) 21.0

    pink, imitation, mix, prepared* (Kool-Aid—regular) 25.0

    pink, imitation, mix, prepared* (Kool-Aid—sugar swt.) 23.0

    pink, imitation, mix, prepared* (Wyler's) 21.0

lemon-lime flavor, mix, prepared* (Kool-Aid) 25.0

lemon-limeade, frozen, reconstituted* (Minute Maid) 26.1

lemon-limeade, frozen, reconstituted* (Snow Crop) 26.1

limeade, frozen, reconstituted* (Minute Maid) 26.8

limeade, frozen, reconstituted* (Snow Crop) 26.8

limeade, imitation, mix, prepared* (Wyler's) 21.0

mixed flavors, canned (Mott's A.M.) 30.4

mixed flavors, canned (Mott's P.M.) 30.4

orange:

    canned (Del Monte) 28.7

    canned (Hi-C) 29.5

    canned (Stokely-Van Camp) 28.5

    dairy-pack (Sealtest) 28.4

    dairy-pack (Sealtest Deluxe) 26.9

    dairy-pack (Tropicana) 26.6

orange flavor:

    mix, prepared* (Knox Gelatin) 28.0

orange flavor, continued

mix, prepared* (Kool-Aid—regular) 25.0
mix, prepared* (Kool-Aid—sugar swt.) 23.0
mix, prepared* (Salada) 23.8
mix, prepared* (Start) 30.0
mix, prepared* (Tang) 29.4
mix, prepared* (Wyler's) 21.0
orangeade, dairy-pack (Sealtest) 31.1
orangeade, frozen, reconstituted* (Minute Maid) 30.3
orangeade, frozen, reconstituted* (Snow Crop) 30.3
orange-apricot, canned (BC) 31.1
orange-apricot, canned (Del Monte) 32.3
orange-banana, canned (BC) 31.1
orange-grapefruit, canned (BC) 31.1
orange-pineapple, canned (BC) 32.7
orange-pineapple, canned (Hi-C) 29.0
peach nectar, canned (Del Monte) 37.9
peach nectar, canned (Heart's Delight) 33.6
pear nectar, canned (Del Monte) 38.4
pear nectar, canned (Heart's Delight) 30.0
pineapple-apricot, canned (Del Monte) 32.6
pineapple-cherry, canned (Del Monte) 24.5
pineapple-grapefruit:
    canned (Del Monte) 31.4
    canned (Dole) 30.8
    canned (Hi-C) 31.4
    canned (Stokely-Van Camp Ping) 29.0
    dairy-pack (Tropicana) 26.6
    pink, canned (Del Monte) 32.3
    pink, canned (Dole) 36.8
pineapple-orange, canned (Del Monte) 31.6
pineapple-orange, canned (Stokely-Van Camp Pong) 27.8
pineapple-pear, canned (Del Monte) 34.0
punch:
    berry, canned (Hawaiian Punch Very Berry) 28.4
    cherry-lemon, frozen, reconstituted* (ReaLemon) 32.0
    fruit, canned (Hawaiian Punch Apple Red) 28.4

punch, continued

fruit, canned (Hawaiian Punch Juicy Red) 28.4
fruit, canned (Hi-C) 32.0
fruit, canned (Mott's Tropical) 30.0
fruit, canned (Stokely-Van Camp) 28.5
fruit, dairy-pack (Tropicana) 26.6
fruit, frozen, reconstituted* (Hawaiian Punch Juicy Red) 28.4
fruit flavor, mix, prepared* (Kool-Aid—regular) 25.0
fruit flavor, mix, prepared* (Kool-Aid—sugar swt.) 23.0
fruit flavor, mix, prepared* (Salada) 24.9
fruit flavor, mix, prepared* (Wyler's) 21.0
grape, canned (Hawaiian Punch) 28.4
grape, canned (Welch's) 32.0
grape, frozen, reconstituted* (Hawaiian Punch) 28.4
grape-lemon, frozen, reconstituted* (ReaLemon) 32.0
lemon-pink, canned (Hawaiian Punch) 28.4
orange, canned (Hawaiian Punch) 28.8
pineapple, canned (Hawaiian Punch) 28.4
pineapple-raspberry, frozen, reconstituted* (ReaLemon) 32.0
raspberry-lemon, frozen, reconstituted* (ReaLemon) 32.0
strawberry-lemon, frozen, reconstituted* (ReaLemon) 32.0
raspberry flavor, mix, prepared* (Kool-Aid—regular) 25.0
raspberry flavor, mix, prepared* (Kool-Aid—sugar swt.) 23.0
raspberry flavor, mix, prepared* (Wyler's) 21.0
strawberry flavor, mix, prepared* (Kool-Aid—regular) 25.0
strawberry flavor, mix, prepared* (Kool-Aid—sugar swt.) 23.0
strawberry flavor, mix, prepared* (Wyler's) 21.0

* *According to package directions*

FRUIT PIE FILLINGS, one whole can or jar*

*See also "Puddings & Custards"
and "Pastry Shells & Pie Crusts"*

	GRAMS
apple:	
(Comstock), 21-oz. can	178.5
(Mott's), 25-oz. can	213.0
(Musselman's), 24-oz. can	206.8
(Stokely-Van Camp), 22-oz. can	142.0
(Wilderness), 21-oz. can	176.0
French (Comstock), 21-oz. can	163.8
apricot (Comstock), 21-oz. can	153.7
blackberry (Comstock), 21-oz. can	212.3
blueberry:	
(Comstock), 21-oz. can	162.3
(Mott's), 25-oz. jar	200.0
(Musselman's), 24-oz. can	208.6
(Stokely-Van Camp), 22-oz. can	179.0
(Wilderness), 21-oz. can	173.0
boysenberry (Comstock), 21-oz. can	160.6
cherry:	
(Comstock), 21-oz. can	165.6
(Mott's), 25-oz. jar	241.0
(Musselman's), 24-oz. can	208.6
(Stokely-Van Camp), 22-oz. can	173.0
(Wilderness), 21-oz. can	170.0
lemon (Comstock), 22-oz. can	180.2
mincemeat:	
(Borden's None Such), 18-oz. jar	234.2
(Comstock), 22-oz. can	196.2
w/rum and brandy (Borden's None Such), 18-oz. jar	223.0
peach (Comstock), 21-oz. can	183.9
peach (Musselman's), 24-oz. can	208.6
peach (Stokely-Van Camp), 22-oz. can	265.0
pineapple (Comstock), 21-oz. can	139.4

Fruit Pie Fillings, continued

pineapple (Wilderness), 21-oz. can 162.0
pumpkin (Comstock), 29.4-oz. can** 165.5
pumpkin (Stokely-Van Camp), 18-oz. can 168.0
raisin (Comstock), 22-oz. can 192.2
raspberry, red (Comstock), 21-oz. can 203.0
strawberry (Comstock), 21-oz. can 155.2

    * *Note variations in size*
** *As prepared for pie*

CHAPTER 2

EGGS, PANCAKES, WAFFLES AND SIMILAR BREAKFAST FOODS

EGGS

See also "Frozen Breakfasts"

	GRAMS
raw*:	
chicken, whole, 1 large	.4
chicken, whole, 1 extra large	.5
chicken, white only, 1 large	tr.
chicken, yolk only, 1 large	.3
duck, whole, 1 large	.6
goose, whole, 1 large	1.8
dried, chicken*:	
whole, 2 tbsp.	.6
white only, 2 tbsp. powder	.8
white only, 2 tbsp. flakes	.7
yolk only, 2 tbsp.	.4
cooked, chicken, one large egg, except as noted:	
boiled*	.4
fried in 1 tbsp. butter*	.4
omelet, plain, made w/milk, cooked in 1 tbsp. butter*	1.5
omelet, cheese, mix (McCormick), 1 serving**	3.0
omelet, mushroom, mix (McCormick), 1 serving**	4.3
omelet, Western, mix (Durkee), 1 serving**	2.2

eggs, cooked, continued

omelet, Western, mix (McCormick), 1 serving** 3.7
poached* 4
scrambled, made w/milk, cooked in 1 tbsp. butter* 1.5
scrambled, mix (Durkee), 1 pkg.† 4.1
scrambled, w/imitation bacon bits, mix (Durkee), 1 pkg.† 6.4

* *Data from United States Department of Agriculture*
** *One-egg omelet, prepared according to package directions*
† *Equals two medium-size eggs, prepared according to package directions*

FROZEN BREAKFASTS, one whole package*

See also "French Toast, Pancakes & Waffles"

	GRAMS
eggs, scrambled, and coffee cake (Swanson), 6½ oz.	26.7
eggs, scrambled, w/link sausage and coffee cake (Swanson), 5½ oz.	17.8
French toast and link sausage (Swanson), 4½ oz.	20.9
pancakes and link sausage (Swanson), 6 oz.	41.6

* *Note variations in size*

FRENCH TOAST, PANCAKES & WAFFLES

See also "Frozen Breakfasts"

	GRAMS
French toast, frozen (Downyflake), 1 slice	15.9
French toast, mix, prepared* (McCormick Batter Mix), 1 slice	19.6
pancakes:	
frozen (Downyflake), 1 cake**	14.7
mix, prepared* (Aunt Jemima), 4"-diameter cake	8.0

pancakes, continued

    mix, prepared* (Aunt Jemima Buckwheat), 4"-diameter cake 8.3
    mix, prepared* (Aunt Jemima Buttermilk), 4"-diameter cake 9.3
    mix, prepared* (Aunt Jemima Easy Pour), 4"-diameter cake 11.0
    mix, prepared* (Duncan Hines Buttermilk), 4"-diameter cake ...19.0
waffles:
    frozen (Aunt Jemima Country), 1 waffle† 8.0
    frozen (Aunt Jemima Original), 1 waffle†† 8.8
    frozen (Downflake), 1 waffle‡ 10.6
    frozen (Downflake), 1 waffle‡‡ 15.3
    mix, prepared* (Aunt Jemima), 4½"-square waffle 22.7
    mix, prepared* (Aunt Jemima Buckwheat), 4½"-square waffle ...23.4
    mix, prepared* (Aunt Jemima Buttermilk), 4½"-square waffle ...20.2
    mix, prepared* (Aunt Jemima Easy Pour), 4½"-square waffle ...26.5

  * *According to package directions*
 ** *From eight-cake/10½-ounce package*
  † *From twelve-waffle/9-ounce package*
 †† *From twelve-waffle/10-ounce package*
  ‡ *From six-waffle/5-ounce package*
 ‡‡ *From ten-waffle/12-ounce package*

CHAPTER 3

CEREALS

CEREAL, COOKED*, one cup, except as noted

See also "Cereal, Ready to Serve"

	GRAMS
barley, pearled (Scotch Brand)	37.0
barley, pearled (Scotch Brand Quick)	49.3
corn:	
grits (Aunt Jemima Hominy—Quick or Regular)	34.5
grits (Quaker Hominy—Quick or Regular)	34.5
grits (Quaker Instant), 1 packet**	17.0
meal mush (Aunt Jemima)	28.5
meal mush (Quaker)	28.5
farina:	
(Cream of Wheat Instant), 1 oz.†	21.2
(Cream of Wheat Mix 'N Eat), 1 packet†	20.8
(Cream of Wheat Quick), 1 oz.†	21.2
(Cream of Wheat Regular), 1 oz.†	21.7
(H-O)	30.0
(Quaker)	22.0
oats:	
(H-O Instant)	28.4
(H-O Old Fashion Oatmeal)	36.0
(H-O Quick)	28.4

oats, continued

(Quaker Instant Oatmeal), 1 packet† 19.0
(Quaker Old Fashioned) 28.5
(Quaker Quick) 28.5
(Ralston Quick) 27.4
(Ralston Regular) 27.4
w/apple and cinnamon (Quaker Instant Oatmeal), 1 packet† 24.0
w/raisin and spice (Quaker Instant Oatmeal), 1 packet† 32.0
oat-wheat (Ralston Wheat Oata) 39.1
rice (Cream of Rice) 31.4
whole wheat (Ralston Instant) 30.4
whole wheat (Ralston Regular) 30.4
whole wheat, rolled (Pettijohns) 31.5

* According to package directions, except as noted
** Dry; approximately one-half cup when cooked
† Dry; approximately three-quarters of a cup when cooked

CEREAL, READY TO SERVE, one cup, except as noted

See also "Cereal, Cooked"

	GRAMS

bran:
(Kellogg's All-Bran) 38.2
(Kellogg's 40% Bran Flakes) 29.5
(Nabisco 100% Bran Flakes) 37.2
(Post 40% Bran Flakes) 31.5
w/raisins (Kellogg's Raisin Bran) 45.0
w/raisins (Post Raisin Bran) 42.0
w/raisins (Raisin Bran Chex) 32.8
w/raisins and cinnamon (Post Cinnamon Raisin Bran) 42.0
w/wheat germ (Kellogg's Bran Buds) 39.8
corn:
(Corn Chex) 19.8
(Kellogg's Corn Flakes) 18.3

corn, continued

(Kellogg's Country Corn Flakes) 18.2
(Kix) 16.0
(Post Toasties Corn Flakes) 24.0
(Ralston Corn Flakes) 24.4
presweetened (Honeycomb Sweet Crisp Corn) 18.8
presweetened (Sugar Frosted Flakes) 33.9
presweetened (Sugar Pops) 25.9
presweetened, cocoa flavor (Cocoa Puffs) 25.0
presweetened, fruit flavor (Trix) 25.2

oats:

(Alpha-Bits) 23.0
(Cheerios) 20.2
(Crispy Critters) 23.0
(Life) 30.0
(Post Fortified Oat Flakes) 28.5
w/marshmallow bits (Lucky Charms) 23.6
presweetened (Frosty O's) 23.9
presweetened (Sugar Jets) 23.7
presweetened, fruit flavor (Froot Loops) 24.5

rice:

(Quaker Puffed Rice) 10.4
(Rice Chex) 22.1
(Rice Krispies) 24.8
presweetened (Frosted Rice Krinkles) 28.6
presweetened (Great Honey Crunchers) 24.8
presweetened (Puffa Puffa Rice) 23.9
presweetened, cocoa flavor (Cocoa Krispies) 25.1
presweetened, orange-honey flavor (Sugar Orange Crisp) 25.0

wheat:

(Grape-Nuts Flakes) 33.0
(Krumbles) 31.7
(Nabisco Shredded Wheat), 1 biscuit 18.7
(Nabisco Spoon Size Shredded Wheat), 1 biscuit 9
(Pep) 23.0
(Quaker Puffed Wheat) 8.3
(Quaker Shredded Wheat), 1 biscuit 15.0

wheat, continued

(Total) 23.1

(Wheat Chex) 35.0

(Wheaties) 23.1

presweetened (Great Honey Crunchers) 23.8

presweetened (Sugar Smacks) 25.0

presweetened (Super Sugar Crisp Puffed Wheat) 28.6

presweetened (Wheat Honeys) 32.6

wheat germ, toasted (Kretschmer) 50.4

wheat germ, toasted, presweetened (Kretschmer Sugar 'N Honey) ..67.6

miscellaneous mixed grains:

(Concentrate) 45.9

(Grape-Nuts) 92.0

(Product 19) 23.0

(Special K) 13.6

(Team Flakes) 18.2

presweetened (Apple Jacks) 25.9

presweetened (Cap'n Crunch) 30.7

presweetened (King Vitaman) 29.3

presweetened (Quake) 23.0

presweetened (Quisp) 19.7

presweetened (Sugar Sparkled Twinkles) 24.2

presweetened, w/berries (Cap'n Crunch's Crunch Berries) 30.7

presweetened, peanut butter flavor
(Cap'n Crunch Peanut Butter) 28.0

CHAPTER 4

BREAD, ROLLS AND OTHER FLOUR PRODUCTS

BREAD, one slice, except as noted
See also "Breads, Sweet," "Breadsticks" and "Rolls & Muffins"

Be careful about comparing the number of carbohydrate grams in commercial, presliced bread. Remember, bread is packaged in different size slices and, to be accurate, you must be certain that you are comparing slices that are equal in size. (See "How to Use This Book," pages 19-23.)

	GRAMS
cheese (Pepperidge Farm Party Slices), 2 slices	5.5
corn and molasses (Pepperidge Farm)	14.4
French, brown and serve, baked (Pepperidge Farm), 1″ slice	15.8
gluten (Thomas' Glutogen)	5.6
Italian, brown and serve, baked (Pepperidge Farm), 1″ slice	16.3
oatmeal (Pepperidge Farm)	12.1
(Profile—dark)	11.0
(Profile—light)	11.3
protein (Thomas' Protogen)	8.7
pumpernickel (Pepperidge Farm Family)	15.8
pumpernickel (Pepperidge Farm Family*)	14.8
pumpernickel (Pepperidge Farm Party Slices), 2 slices	7.7
rye:	
(Pepperidge Farm Family)	15.7

rye, continued

(Pepperidge Farm Family*) 14.7
(Pepperidge Farm Party Slices), 2 slices 6.0
(Pepperidge Farm Seedless) 15.5
(Pepperidge Farm Seedless*) 14.5
(Wonder) 10.5
(Wonder Beefsteak) 15.6
(Wonder Beefsteak Family) 11.7

wheat:

(Buttertop Home Pride) 11.5
(Pepperidge Farm Sprouted Wheat) 11.3
(Pepperidge Farm Whole Wheat) 11.4
(Thomas' Whole Wheat) 11.2
(Wonder Golden Wheat) 12.1
(Wonder 100% Whole Wheat) 11.4
cracked wheat (Pepperidge Farm) 12.8
cracked wheat, honey (Wonder) 11.3
honey (Pepperidge Farm Honey Wheatberry) 15.4

wheat germ (Pepperidge Farm) 11.4

white:

(Buttertop Home Pride) 13.2
(Daffodil Farm) 11.3
(Pepperidge Farm English Tea Loaf) 12.0
(Pepperidge Farm Large) 13.1
(Pepperidge Farm Large**) 11.4
(Pepperidge Farm Sandwich) 11.5
(Pepperidge Farm Sandwich*) 10.5
(Pepperidge Farm Toasting) 15.6
(Pepperidge Farm Very Thin†) 7.4
(Pepperidge Farm Very Thin††) 8.0
(Thomas') 12.2
(Wonder) 12.6

* Florida distribution only
** California distribution only
† Eastern distribution only
†† Midwestern distribution only

BREADS, SWEET, one slice, except as noted

See also "Muffins, Sweet"

	GRAMS
banana nut, canned ((Dromedary), ½" slice*	12.3
brown, canned (B & M), ½" slice*	16.6
brown, w/raisins, canned (B & M), ½" slice*	16.6
chocolate nut, canned (Crosse & Blackwell), ½" slice*	14.9
chocolate nut, canned (Dromedary), ½" slice*	14.5
cinnamon raisin (Pepperidge Farm)	13.6
cinnamon raisin (Thomas')	12.2
cinnamon raisin (Wonder)	13.1
corn, mix, prepared** (Aunt Jemima), 1 slice†	15.0
corn, mix, prepared** (Dromedary), 2" x 2" slice	18.5
date nut (Thomas')	18.0
date nut, canned (Dromedary), ½" slice*	12.2
fruit and nut, canned (Crosse & Blackwell), ½" slice*	13.6
orange nut, canned (Crosse & Blackwell), ½" slice*	15.5
orange nut, canned (Dromedary), ½" slice*	13.4
spice nut, canned (Crosse & Blackwell), ½" slice*	13.3

* *Approximately one ounce*
** *According to package directions*
† *One-twelfth of whole bread*

BREADSTICKS, one piece

	GRAMS
plain (Stella D'Oro)	6.6
onion flavor (Stella D'Oro)	6.8
w/sesame seeds (Stella D'Oro)	5.7

ROLLS & MUFFINS, one piece

See also "Muffins, Sweet"

To compare the carbohydrate gram content of different brands
and types of commercial rolls and muffins, you should be
certain you are comparing products that are the same size.
Otherwise, your comparisons are likely to be inaccurate. (See
"How to Use This Book," pages 19-23.)

GRAMS

biscuits, refrigerator, baked (Pillsbury Buttermilk) 10.7
biscuits, refrigerator, baked (Pillsbury Flaky Baking Powder) 7.9
biscuits, refrigerator, baked (Pillsbury Hungry Jack) 10.9
muffins, English (Pepperidge Farm) 27.6
muffins, English (Thomas') 28.7
muffins, English (Wonder) 26.7
popovers, mix, prepared* (Flako), 3½" x 3" diameter 22.0
rolls, hard, brown and serve, baked:
   (Pepperidge Farm Club) 23.3
   (Pepperidge Farm Triple French; 3-oz. size) 51.4
   (Pepperidge Farm Twin French; 5-oz. size) 75.7
   (Pepperidge Farm Hearth) 11.6
   (Wonder) 13.9
   w/sesame seeds (Pepperidge Farm Sesame Crisp)** 13.1
   w/sesame seeds (Pepperidge Farm Sesame Crisp)† 12.3
rolls, soft, ready to serve:
   (Pepperidge Farm Butter Crescent) 13.2
   (Pepperidge Farm Butterfly) 7.9
   (Pepperidge Farm Dinner) 9.9
   (Pepperidge Farm Old Fashioned) 7.6
   (Pepperidge Farm Party Pan—Finger) 9.2
   (Pepperidge Farm Party Pan—Round) 5.5
   frankfurter (Pepperidge Farm) 19.3
   frankfurter (Wonder) 21.3
   hamburger (Pepperidge Farm) 18.9

rolls, soft, ready to serve, continued

    hamburger (Pepperidge Farm)†† 19.5

    hamburger (Wonder) 21.3

rolls, soft, baked or heated:

    brown and serve (Pepperidge Farm Golden Twist) 14.0

    frozen (Sara Lee Finger) 10.5

    frozen (Sara Lee Parkerhouse) 10.5

    frozen (Sara Lee Sesame Seed) 10.5

    refrigerator (Pillsbury Butterflake) 8.8

    refrigerator (Pillsbury Crescent) 13.0

    refrigerator (Pillsbury Parkerhouse) 10.6

    refrigerator (Pillsbury Snowflake) 8.8

   * *According to package directions*
  ** *Eastern distribution only*
   † *Midwest distribution only*
  †† *California distribution only*

MUFFINS, SWEET, one piece

See also "Breads, Sweet," "Specialty Snack Cakes"
and "Coffee Cakes & Other Sweet Baked Goods"

When comparing the number of carbohydrate grams in different brands and types of commercial sweet muffins, be sure you are comparing products that are the same size. If you're not sure, don't make comparisons as they are likely to be inaccurate. (See "How to Use This Book," pages 19-23.)

                                        GRAMS

blueberry, frozen (Howard Johnson Toastees) 16.7

blueberry, frozen (Morton) 20.8

blueberry, mix, prepared* (Duncan Hines), 1 medium** 16.0

bran (Thomas' Toast-r-Cakes) 17.1

cinnamon, frozen (Aunt Jemima Sticks) 21.0

cinnamon raisin, frozen (Howard Johnson Toastees) 19.1

Muffins, Sweet, continued

corn:

(Drake's) 33.7
(Thomas') 25.8
frozen (Aunt Jemima Sticks) 27.0
frozen (Howard Johnson Toastees) 20.4
frozen (Morton) 20.4
mix, prepared* (Dromedary), 2½" diameter 20.5
mix, prepared* (Flako), 1⅜" x 2½" diameter 21.0
orange, frozen (Howard Johnson Toastees) 16.4
raisin (Drake's Raisin Snack) 38.2
raisin (Wonder Rounds) 30.3
raisin (Wonder Scones) 27.9

* *According to package directions*
** *Approximately 1.2-oz. muffin*

CRUMBS, MEAL & STUFFINGS, four ounces

	GRAMS
crumbs, bread (Wonder)	81.9
crumbs, bread, flavored (La Rosa)	79.9
crumbs, graham cracker (Nabisco)	87.1

meal:

cracker (Keebler)	91.4
cracker, salted (Nabisco)	87.4
cracker, unsalted (Nabisco)	90.4
graham cracker (Keebler)	85.5
matzo (Manischewitz)	94.0
stuffing, corn bread (Pepperidge Farm)	83.6
stuffing, cube bread (Pepperidge Farm)	63.0
stuffing, herb-seasoned bread (Pepperidge Farm)	89.4

SEASONED COATING MIXES, one envelope

See also "Seasoning & Roasting Mixes"

	GRAMS
for chicken (Shake 'n Bake)	40.0
for fish (Shake 'n Bake)	33.0
for hamburger (Shake 'n Bake)	31.6
for pork (Shake 'n Bake)	46.3

FLOUR*, four ounces**

	GRAMS
buckwheat, dark	81.6
buckwheat, light	90.2
carob (St. Johnsbread)	91.5
corn	87.1
rye, dark	77.2
rye, light	88.3
rye, medium	84.8
wheat:	
all purpose	86.3
bread	84.7
cake or pastry	90.0
gluten	53.5
self-rising	84.1
whole grain	80.5

 * *Data from United States Department of Agriculture*
** *Approximately one cup, sifted*

CHAPTER 5

CRACKERS

CRACKERS, one piece

See also "Cracker Sandwiches"

Bear in mind that crackers are available in dozens of sizes and shapes; therefore it is hard—indeed, often impossible—to accurately compare the carbohydrate content of different brands and types. (See "How to Use This Book," pages 19-23.)

	GRAMS
(American Harvest)	2.0
arrowroot, see "Cookies," page 173	
bacon flavor (Keebler Bacon Toast)	1.9
bacon flavor (Nabisco Bacon Thins)	1.2
butter flavor:	
(Hi-Ho)	2.0
(Keebler Butter Thins)	2.8
(Keebler Club)	2.1
(Keebler Townhouse)	2.0
(Nabisco Butter Thins)	2.4
(Ritz)	2.1
(Tam-Tams)	1.7
butter-cheese flavor (Ritz Cheese)	1.9
butter-sesame (Nabisco)	1.9

Crackers, continued
cheese flavor:
(Cheese Nips) 7
(Cheese Tid-Bits) 6
(Cheez-It) 6
(Che-Zo) 6
(Keebler Cheese Toast) 1.9
(Pepperidge Farm Cheddar Goldfish) 3
(Pepperidge Farm Parmesan Goldfish) 3
chicken flavor (Chicken In A Biskit) 1.2
graham crackers, see "Cookies," page 177
matzo, one sheet:
(Horowitz-Margareten Oven Crisp) 28.3
(Manischewitz American) 22.8
(Manischewitz Egg) 26.5
(Manischewitz Egg 'N Onion) 24.0
(Manischewitz Regular) 26.9
(Manischewitz Tasteas) 23.6
(Manischewitz Thin Teas) 24.3
(Manischewitz Whole Wheat) 24.2
onion flavor:
(Keebler Toast) 2.0
(Manischewitz Tams) 1.9
(Meal Mates Bread Wafers) 3.4
(Nabisco French) 1.6
(Pepperidge Farm Goldfish) 4
oyster (Dandy) 5
oyster (Oysterettes) 6
oyster (Sunshine) 7
pizza flavor (Pepperidge Farm Goldfish) 4
potato flavor (Chippers) 1.8
rye:
(Keebler Rye Toast) 2.3
(Meal Mates Bread Wafers) 3.4
(Rye Crispbread) 5.5
(Ry-Krisp) 4.8
seasoned (Ry-Krisp) 4.5

saltines, soda and water crackers:
  (Crown Pilot) 12.4
  (Escort) 2.7
  (Huntley & Palmers Fortts' Oliver) 6.0
  (Jacob's Biscuits for Cheese) 6.0
  (Jacob's English Cream Crackers) 19.0
  (Jacob's Golden Puffs) 6.0
  (Jacob's Large Water Biscuits) 6.0
  (Keebler Milk Lunch) 4.5
  (Keebler Sea Toast) 10.9
  (Krispy) 2.0
  (Krispy—unsalted) 2.1
  (Pepperidge Farm Lightly Salted Goldfish) 4
  (Premium) 2.0
  (Premium—unsalted) 2.0
  (Royal Lunch) 7.9
  (Waldorf Low-Sodium) 2.4
  (Zesta) 2.0
sesame bread wafers (Keebler) 2.0
sesame bread wafers (Meal Mates) 2.9
sesame-butter flavor (Nabisco) 1.9
sesame-cheese flavor (Sunshine Sesame Cheese Snacks) 2.2
sesame-garlic flavor (Pepperidge Farm Goldfish) 4
(Sociables) 1.3
toasted crackers:
  (Dutch Rusk) 10.5
  (Holland Rusk) 9.0
  (Nabisco Zwieback) 5.4
  (Sunshine Toasted Wafers) 1.2
  (Sunshine Zwieback) 5.3
  (Uneeda) 3.7
(Triangle Thins) 1.1
(Waverly) 2.6
wheat:
  (Jacob's Goldgrain) 6.0
  (Keebler Wheat Toast) 1.9

wheat crackers, continued

    (Nabisco Wheat Thins) 1.2
    (Triscuit) 3.0

CRACKER SANDWICHES, one piece

See also "Crackers"

Remember that cracker sandwiches come in a variety of sizes and shapes; therefore, it is difficult to accurately compare the carbohydrate gram content of different brands and types. (See "How to Use This Book," pages 19-23.)

	GRAMS
cheese and cheese flavor:	
(Cheesewich)	1.9
(Cheez Waffies)	1.9
(Huntley & Palmers)	12.0
(Nabisco)	3.1
(Nab Cheese on Rye)	2.9
(Wise Cheese-N-Cheese)	3.8
cheese-bacon flavor (Nab Cheese 'n Bacon)	3.1
cheese-peanut butter:	
(Nab—squares; 4-piece/1-oz. pkg.)	3.7
(Nab—squares; 6-piece/1½-oz. pkg.)	3.4
(Nab—squares; 6-piece/1¾-oz. pkg.)	4.3
(Nab—variety pack; 6-piece/1½-oz. pkg.)	2.8
(Nab—variety pack; 6-piece/1¾-oz. pkg.)	3.4
(O-So-Gud)	4.1
(Wise)	3.5
malted milk-peanut butter (Nab; 4-piece/1-oz. pkg.)	4.0
malted milk-peanut butter (Nab; 6-piece/1⅜-oz. pkg.)	3.7
peanut butter (Adora)	4.5
peanut butter (Bana-Bee)	5.2
peanut butter (Wise Peanut Butter Toast)	3.7

CHAPTER 6

CHEESE AND CHEESE PRODUCTS

CHEESE, one ounce, except as noted

See also "Grated & Shredded Cheese," "Cheese Foods" and "Cheese Spreads"

Unless otherwise noted, the figure listed for any cheese in this category applies to all forms in which it may be packaged— sliced, in bars, loaves, wedges, etc. For example, Kraft's Old English cheese is packaged in loaves and slices, but in either form it contains the same .5 carbohydrate grams per ounce. However, do be careful not to confuse cheese with a cheese *spread* or a cheese *food* that bears the same or a similar name. For instance, in addition to Old English cheese, you can also buy Old English cheese spread, which contains .6 carbohydrate grams per ounce. Generally, it isn't hard to differentiate between cheese and cheese spreads, but cheese foods sometimes pose a problem (especially when they are packaged in slices). Check the label if you're confused about a product; if it is a cheese spread or a cheese food, the label will say so.

GRAMS

American:
natural (Kraft)	.6
processed (Borden)	.6
processed (Borden Made in Wisconsin)	.6

American, continued

   processed (Kraft) 5
   processed (Sealtest) 5
   sharp, processed (Kraft Old English) 5
   sharp, processed (Vera-Sharp) 6
asiago (Frigo) 6
blue:
   (Blue Chip Brand) 5
   (Blufort Brand), 1¼-oz. portion 7
   (Borden Danish) 6
   (Flora Danica) 6
   (Foremost Blue Moon) 6
   (Frigo) 5
   (Kraft) 5
(Bonbel Brand) 5
bondost (Kraft) 4
brick:
   natural (Borden) 5
   natural (Kraft) 3
   natural, aged (Lager-Käse) 3
   processed (Kraft) 4
Camembert (Borden) 5
Camembert (Kraft Tiny Dane) 5
caraway (Kraft) 6
(Chantelle Brand) 3
cheddar:
   (Borden) 6
   (Borden Longhorn) 6
   (Borden Wisconsin Old Fashioned) 6
   (Coon Brand) 6
   (Cracker Barrel Brand) 6
   (Kraft) 6
   (Kraft Longhorn) 6
   (Kraft Midget Horn) 6
   (Martin's Rabbit Brand) 6
   (Sealtest) 6

Cheese, continued

colby:
(Borden) 6
(Cracker Barrel Brand) 6
(Jay Brand) 6
(Kraft) 6
(Kraft Longhorn) 6
cottage, see "Cottage Cheese," pages 67-68
cream, see "Cream & Neufchâtel Cheese," pages 65-66
Edam:
(House of Gold) 3
(Kraft) 3
(Kraft Domestic) 3
(Kraft Imported Holland) 3
farmer (Breakstone Midget) 8
fontina (Kraft) 6
Frankenmuth (Kraft) 7
Gjetost goat cheese (Kraft) 13.0
Gorgonzola (Kraft) 4
Gouda (Borden Dutch Maid) 5
Gouda (Jay Brand) 5
Gouda (Kraft) 5
Gruyère (Borden) 5
Gruyère (Kraft Imported Switzerland Crown Brand) 6
Gruyère (Swiss Knight) 5
jack-dry (Kraft) 4
jack-fresh (Kraft) 4
Leyden (Kraft) 7
(Liederkranz Brand) 3
Limburger:
(Borden Dutch Maid) 6
(Kraft) 6
(Mohawk Valley Brand) 6
(Moose Brand) 6
Monterey Jack (Borden) 6
Monterey Jack (Frigo) 4
Monterey Jack (Kraft) 4

Cheese, continued

Mozzarella:

(Borden) 8

(Dorman's) 5

(Frigo) 3

(Kraft) 3

Muenster:

natural (Borden) 7

natural (Dorman's) 2

natural (Kraft) 3

processed (Kraft) 6

Neufchâtel, see "Cream & Neufchâtel Cheese," pages 66-67

nuworld (Kraft) 7

Parmesan (Frigo) 8

Parmesan (Kraft) 8

Pepato (Frigo) 8

pimento (Borden) 5

pimento (Borden Made in Wisconsin) 5

pimento (Kraft) 4

Pinconning (Kraft) 7

pizza (Borden) 8

pizza (Frigo) 3

pizza (Kraft) 3

Port Salut (Dorman's) 1

Port Salut (Kraft) 3

Primost (Kraft) 13.0

Provolone (Borden) 1.0

Provolone (Frigo) 5

Provolone (Kraft) 5

Ricotta (Borden) 1.0

Ricotta (Breakstone) 1.3

Ricotta (Frigo) 1.1

Romano (Borden Italian Pecorino) 8

Romano (Frigo) 8

Romano (Kraft) 8

Roquefort (Borden Napoleon Brand) 6

Roquefort (Kraft Imported Louis Rigal) 5

Cheese, continued

sage (Kraft) 6
Sapsago (Kraft) 1.7
Sardo Romano (Kraft) 8
Scamorze (Frigo) 3
Scamorze (Kraft) 3
Swiss:
  natural (Borden) 5
  natural (Borden Imported Finland) 5
  natural (Borden Imported Switzerland) 5
  natural (Dorman's) 3
  natural (Dorman's Austrian) 2
  natural (Kraft) 5
  natural (Kraft Imported Finland) 5
  natural (Kraft Imported Switzerland) 5
  natural (Sealtest) 5
  processed (Borden) 5
  processed (Borden Made in Wisconsin) 5
  processed (Kraft—loaf) 5
  processed (Kraft—slices) 6
  processed (Milkboy Brand) 5
  hickory smoke flavor (Borden) 5
  w/Muenster (Kraft) 6
Tilsiter (Dorman's) 2
washed curd (Kraft) 6

GRATED & SHREDDED CHEESE, one tablespoon

See also "Cheese" and "Cheese Spreads"

	GRAMS
American, grated (Borden)	2.6
American, grated (Kraft)	2.0
cheddar, shredded (Cracker Barrel Brand)	.2
Mozzarella, shredded (Kraft)	.1

Grated & Shredded Cheese, continued

Parmesan:

grated (Borden) 1

grated (Frigo) 2

grated (Kraft) 2

grated (La Rosa) 1

shredded (Kraft) 2

Parmesan-Romano, grated (Borden) 1

Parmesan-Romano, grated (Kraft) 2

pizza, shredded (Kraft) 1

Romano, grated (Frigo) 2

Romano, grated (Kraft) 2

Romano, shredded (Kraft) 2

Romano-Parmesan:

grated (Kraft) 2

bacon-smoke flavor, grated (Kraft) 2

garlic flavor, grated (Kraft) 2

onion flavor, grated (Kraft) 2

CHEESE FOODS*, one ounce

See also "Cheese" and "Cheese Spreads"

	GRAMS
American (Borden)	2.0
American (Kraft)	2.4
w/bacon (Kraft Cheez'n Bacon)	.7
w/bacon (Kraft Handi-Snack Links)	2.2
w/garlic (Kraft Handi-Snack Links)	2.2
hickory smoke flavor (Kraft Smokelle Handi-Snack Links)	2.2
w/jalapeno pepper and pimento (Kraft Handi-Snack Links)	2.2
(Kraft Munst-ett)	1.7
(Kraft Superblend)	1.6
pimento (Borden)	2.0
pimento (Kraft)	2.5

Cheese Foods, continued

pizza flavor (Kraft Pizzalone) 5
w/salami (Nippy Brand Handi-Snack Links) 2.2
Swiss (Borden) 2.0
Swiss (Kraft) 2.3
Swiss (Kraft Handi-Snack Links) 1.4

* See "Cheese," page 58, to be certain you don't confuse a cheese food with cheese or a cheese spread

CHEESE SPREADS*, one ounce

See also "Cream & Neufchâtel Cheese" and "Cheese Foods"

	GRAMS
American (Kraft)	1.7
American (Snack Mate)	2.3
w/bacon (Borden Cheese 'N Bacon)	1.2
w/bacon (Kraft)	.6
w/bacon (Kraft Squeez-A-Snak)	.5
blue (Borden Blue Brand)	2.3
blue (Borden Vera Blue)	.6
blue (Wispride)	3.1
cheddar (Snack Mate)	2.3
cheddar, seasoned (Snack Mate)	2.7
cheddar, sharp (Wispride)	2.9
(Cheez Whiz)	1.7
w/garlic (Borden)	2.3
w/garlic (Kraft)	2.2
w/garlic (Kraft Squeez-A-Snak)	.6
hickory smoke flavor (Borden)	1.3
hickory smoke flavor (Kraft Smokelle)	.5
hickory smoke flavor (Kraft Squeez-A-Snak)	.5
hickory smoke flavor (Snack Mate)	2.7
imitation (Kraft Tasty Loaf)	3.6
w/jalapeno pepper and pimento (Cheez Whiz Jalapeno Pepper)	1.9

Cheese Spreads, continued

(Laughing Cow) 1.0
limburger (Borden) 2.3
limburger (Mohawk Valley Brand) 3
limburger (Moose Brand) 3
onion, French (Snack Mate) 2.4
pimento:
    (Cheez Whiz Pimento) 1.7
    (Kraft) 2.3
    (Kraft Squeez-A-Snak) 6
    (Sealtest) 1.7
    (Snack Mate) 2.2
    (Velveeta Pimento) 2.6
sharp:
    (Kraft Old English) 6
    (Kraft Sharpie) 5
    (Kraft Squeez-A-Snak) 6
    (Vera-Sharp) 1.3
Swiss (Kraft) 5
(Velveeta) 2.6

* *See "Cheese," page 58, to be certain you don't confuse a cheese spread with cheese or a cheese food*

CREAM & NEUFCHÂTEL CHEESE, one ounce

See also "Cheese Spreads" and "Dips, Ready to Serve"

                                                 GRAMS

cream cheese:
    plain (Borden) 6
    plain (Breakstone) 6
    plain (Kraft) 6
    plain (Philadelphia Brand) 9
    plain (Sealtest) 6
    w/chive (Borden) 6

Cream Cheese, continued

w/chive (Kraft) 8
w/chive (Philadelphia Brand) 8
w/olive and pimento (Kraft) 8
w/pimento (Borden) 6
w/pimento (Kraft) 7
w/pimento (Philadelphia Brand) 7
w/pineapple (Kraft) 2.5
w/Roquefort cheese (Kraft) 7
cream cheese, imitation (Philadelphia Brand) 2.0
cream cheese, imitation (Velva Creme) 9
cream cheese, whipped:
  plain (Temp-Tee) 6
  w/bacon and horseradish (Kraft) 7
  w/blue cheese (Kraft) 1.2
  w/chive (Kraft) 1.0
  w/herbs and spices (Kraft Catalina) 1.1
  w/onion (Kraft) 1.5
  w/pimento (Kraft) 1.2
  w/salami (Kraft) 1.2
  w/smoked salmon (Kraft) 1.7
Neufchâtel cheese:
  plain (Borden Eagle Brand) 8
  plain (Kraft) 7
  w/bacon and horseradish (Kraft Party Snack) 7
  w/blue cheese (Kraft Roka Brand) 6
  w/chipped beef (Kraft Party Snack) 1.2
  w/chive (Kraft Party Snack) 8
  w/clam (Kraft Party Snack) 8
  w/olive and pimento (Borden) 2.7
  w/olive and pimento (Kraft) 1.2
  w/onion (Kraft Party Snack) 1.6
  w/pimento (Borden) 2.9
  w/pimento (Kraft) 1.4
  w/pimento (Kraft Party Snack) 1.4
  w/pineapple (Borden) 3.1

Neufchâtel cheese, continued

w/pineapple (Kraft) 2.7
w/relish (Borden) 3.5
w/relish (Kraft) 3.3

COTTAGE CHEESE, half cup

GRAMS

creamed:
   (Borden) 3.3
   (Breakstone) 2.8
   (Breakstone California Style) 3.0
   (Breakstone Low Fat) 3.0
   (Breakstone Tiny Soft Curd) 3.0
   (Foremost) 2.7
   (Light n' Lively) 3.6
   (Meadow Gold) 3.0
   (Pet) 3.5
   (Sealtest) 2.4
   (Sealtest Lowfat) 3.6
creamed, flavored:
   w/chive (Borden) 3.3
   w/chive (Breakstone) 3.0
   w/chive (Sealtest) 2.4
   w/chive-pepper (Sealtest) 2.7
   w/peach-pineapple (Sealtest) 9.0
   w/pineapple (Borden) 8.4
   w/pineapple (Breakstone) 3.0
   w/pineapple (Sealtest) 8.0
   w/vegetable salad (Borden) 4.7
   w/vegetable salad (Sealtest Spring Garden) 3.4
creamed partially:
   (Foremost So-Lo) 3.2
   (Light n' Lively) 2.8

cottage cheese, creamed partially, continued

(Meadow Gold) 3.0
(Pet) 3.2
uncreamed (Breakstone Pot Style) 1.9
uncreamed (Breakstone Skim Milk) 2.2
uncreamed (Sealtest Dry) 8

WELSH RAREBIT, one cup

	GRAMS
canned (Snow's)	16.8
w/sherry, canned (Snow's)	16.8

CHAPTER 7

YOGURT
AND SOUR CREAM

YOGURT, eight-ounce cup, except as noted

	GRAMS
plain:	
(Borden Swiss Style)	14.0
(Breakstone)	13.4
(Dannon)	12.4
(Light n' Lively) 8 oz.*	16.8
(Pet)	12.2
(Yami), 8 oz.*	12.8
apple:	
cinnamon (Breakstone)	53.2
Dutch (Dannon)	41.9
spiced (Borden Swiss Style)	45.3
spiced (Light n' Lively), 8 oz.*	47.2
spiced (Meadow Gold Western Style), 8 oz.*	54.0
spiced (Yami), 8 oz.*	38.8
apricot:	
(Borden Swiss Style)	45.3
(Breakstone)	54.0
(Dannon)	41.9
(Yami), 8 oz.*	38.8
blueberry:	
(Borden Swiss Style)	45.3

blueberry, continued

   (Breakstone) 53.2

   (Breakstone Swiss Parfait) 56.8

   (Dannon) 41.9

   (Dannon "Danny"), 4-fl.-oz. carton 21.0

   (Light n' Lively), 8 oz.* 50.6

   (Meadow Gold Swiss Style), 8 oz.* 49.0

   (Meadow Gold Western Style), 8 oz.* 54.0

   (Sanna Swiss Miss), 4-fl.-oz. carton 19.0

   (Yami), 8 oz.* 38.8

blackberry (Yami), 8 oz.* 38.8

boysenberry:

   (Borden Swiss Style) 45.3

   (Dannon) 41.9

   (Meadow Gold Western Style), 8 oz.* 54.0

   (Yami), 8 oz.* 38.8

cherry:

   (Borden Swiss Style) 45.3

   (Dannon) 41.9

   (Meadow Gold Western Style), 8 oz.* 54.0

   (Yami), 8 oz.* 38.8

   black (Breakstone Swiss Parfait), 5-fl.-oz. carton 34.6

cherry-vanilla (Borden Swiss Style) 45.3

coffee (Borden Swiss Style) 45.3

coffee (Dannon) 26.7

cranberry-orange (Borden Swiss Style) 45.3

fruit cup (Dannon) 41.9

lemon (Light n' Lively), 8 oz.* 43.4

lemon (Yami), 8 oz.* 38.8

lime (Borden Swiss Style) 45.3

orange, Mandarin:

   (Borden Swiss Style) 49.7

   (Breakstone Swiss Parfait) 57.4

   (Breakstone Swiss Parfait), 5-fl.-oz. carton 35.8

   (Meadow Gold Western Style), 8 oz.* 54.0

   (Yami), 8 oz.* 38.8

Yogurt, continued

peach:

    (Borden Swiss Style) 48.2

    (Breakstone Swiss Parfait) 53.7

    (Light n' Lively), 8 oz.* 49.3

    (Meadow Gold Western Style), 8 oz.* 54.0

    (Yami), 8 oz.* 38.8

    Melba (Breakstone Swiss Parfait), 5-fl.-oz. carton 37.7

pear (Borden Swiss Style) 45.3

pineapple:

    (Breakstone) 54.0

    (Light n' Lively), 8 oz.* 47.2

    (Meadow Gold Western Style), 8 oz.* 54.0

    (Yami), 8 oz.* 38.8

pineapple-orange (Dannon) 41.9

pineapple-orange, w/orange coating, frozen
    (Dannon Danny-on-a-Stick), 2½-fl.-oz. bar 11.4

prune:

    (Borden Swiss Style) 45.3

    (Breakstone) 53.2

    (Dannon) 41.9

    (Light n' Lively), 8 oz.* 50.8

    (Yami), 8 oz.* 38.8

raspberry:

    (Borden Swiss Style) 45.3

    (Breakstone) 53.2

    (Breakstone Swiss Parfait) 54.4

    (Dannon) 41.9

    (Dannon "Danny"), 4-fl.-oz. carton 21.0

    (Light n' Lively), 8 oz.* 41.8

    (Meadow Gold Swiss Style), 8 oz.* 49.0

    (Sanna Swiss Miss), 4-fl.-oz. carton 19.0

    (Yami), 8 oz.* 38.8

    w/chocolate coating, frozen
        (Dannon Danny-on-a-Stick), 2½-fl.-oz. bar 14.5

strawberry:

    (Borden Swiss Style) 48.2

strawberry yogurt, continued

(Breakstone) 53.7
(Breakstone Swiss Parfait) 54.1
(Breakstone Swiss Parfait), 5-fl.-oz. carton 33.6
(Dannon) 41.9
(Dannon "Danny"), 4-fl.-oz. carton 21.0
(Light n' Lively), 8 oz.* 44.3
(Meadow Gold Swiss Style), 8 oz.* 49.0
(Meadow Gold Western Style), 8 oz.* 54.0
(Sanna Swiss Miss), 4-fl.-oz. carton 19.0
(Yami), 8 oz.* 38.8
w/chocolate coating, frozen
   (Dannon Danny-on-a-Stick), 2½-fl.-oz. bar 14.5

vanilla:

(Borden Swiss Style) 49.2
(Breakstone) 30.6
(Dannon) 26.7
(Light n' Lively), 8 oz.* 32.7
(Yami), 8 oz.* 22.6

* *Net weight; volume is approximately seven-eighths of a cup*

SOUR CREAM, one tablespoon

	GRAMS
plain:	
(Borden Dairy Maid)	.5
(Breakstone)	.5
(Foremost)	.6
(Meadow Gold)	.5
(Pet)	.6
(Sealtest)	.5
half and half, 10.5% fat (Foremost)	.6
half and half, 12.0% fat (Foremost)	.6
half and half, 12.0% fat (Sealtest)	.5

CHAPTER 8

DIPS, APPETIZERS
AND HORS D'OEUVRES

DIPS, READY TO SERVE,
eight-ounce container, except as noted

See also "Dip Mixes"

	GRAMS
bacon and horseradish (Borden), 4-oz. carton	11.6
bacon and horseradish (Kraft Ready)	6.6
bacon and horseradish (Kraft Teez)	12.7
bacon and smoke flavor (Sealtest Dip 'n Dressing)	13.9
blue cheese (Kraft Ready)	12.5
blue cheese (Kraft Teez)	10.7
blue cheese (Sealtest Dip 'n Dressing)	12.1
chipped beef (Sealtest Dip 'n Dressing)	14.6
clam (Kraft Ready)	19.5
clam (Kraft Teez)	12.2
clam and lobster (Borden), 4-oz. carton	6.8
dill pickle (Kraft Ready)	14.5
garden spice (Borden), 4-oz. carton	8.4
garlic (Kraft Teez)	11.8
green chili (Borden)	17.0
green goddess (Kraft Teez)	12.0
jalapeno bean (Fritos), 10½-oz. can	38.1
jalapeno bean (Old El Paso), 7½-oz. can	52.5

Dips, Ready to Serve, continued

onion (Kraft Ready) 15.6
onion, French (Borden), 4-oz. carton 10.0
onion, French (Borden—sour cream base) 20.1
onion, French (Kraft Teez) 12.0
onion, French (Sealtest Dip 'n Dressing) 17.2
onion and garlic (Sealtest Dip 'n Dressing) 17.9
(Sealtest Casino Dip 'n Dressing) 16.7

DIP MIXES, one packet*

See also "Dips, Ready-to-Eat"

To determine the carbohydrate gram content of a prepared dip mix, simply combine the number of grams in the dry mix with the number of grams in the ingredient(s) you add to it—for example, a cup of sour cream or four ounces of cream cheese. When the dip is prepared, take careful note of its volume (two cups, one and a half cups, etc.) and you'll be able to determine the carbohydrate content of an individual serving.

	GRAMS
bacon-onion (Fritos), 0.56 oz.	6.9
barbecue (Salada Bar-B-Q), 1 oz.	8.2
bleu cheese (Fritos), 0.56 oz.	4.6
cheddar and sesame (Salada), 1 oz.	7.3
chili con queso (Fritos), 0.56 oz.	7.1
dill and chive (Salada), 1 oz.	8.5
garlic and onion (McCormick), 1¼ oz.	12.0
horseradish, w/imitation bacon bits (McCormick), 1¼ oz.	9.0
onion:	
(Knorr Swiss Soup-Dip), 2 oz.	34.0
(Lipton Soup-Dip), 1⅜ oz.	22.1
(Wyler's Soup-Dip), 1¼ oz.	28.0
French (Salada), 1 oz.	8.7
green (Fritos), 0.56 oz.	10.6

onion, continued

    green (Lawry's), 0.56 oz. 8.3
    toasted (Fritos), 0.56 oz. 9.8
    toasted (Lawry's), 0.56 oz. 8.6
    toasted (McCormick), 1¼ oz. 12.0
onion and garlic (Salada), 1 oz. 8.2
taco (Fritos), 0.56 oz. 9.5

* *Note variations in size*

APPETIZERS, HORS D'OEUVRES & SNACKS, FROZEN

*See also "Appetizers, Hors d'Oeuvres & Snacks,
Canned, Dried and in Jars"*

                                                                         GRAMS

burrito rolls:
    bean and bacon (Patio), ½-oz. roll 4.4
    beef (Patio), ½-oz. roll 4.0
    chicken (Patio), ½-oz. roll 4.5
cheese straws (Durkee), 1 straw* 1.2
egg rolls:
    chicken (Chun King), ½-oz. roll 3.2
    chicken and mushroom (Mow Sang), 1-oz. roll 7.0
    meat (Chun King), 1-oz. roll 7.8
    meat and lobster (Chun King), ½-oz. roll 3.7
    meat and shrimp (Chun King), ½-oz. roll 3.7
    meat and shrimp (Chun King), 1-oz. roll 5.8
    pork, barbecue (Mow Sang), 1-oz. roll 6.0
    shrimp (Chun King), ½-oz. roll 3.8
    shrimp (Chun King), 1-oz. roll 7.6
    shrimp (Mow Sang), 1-oz. roll 6.0
    shrimp (Temple), 2½-oz. roll 15.4
    vegetable (Mow Sang), 1-oz. roll 7.0
franks "in blankets" (Durkee Franks-N-Blanket), 1 frank** 1.0

Appetizers, Hors d'Oeuvres & Snacks, Frozen, continued

pizza rolls:

    cheeseburger (Jeno's), ½-oz. roll 3.9

    pepperoni (Jeno's), ½-oz. roll 3.8

    sausage (Jeno's), ½-oz. roll 3.8

    shrimp (Jeno's), ½-oz. roll 3.5

    Sloppy Joe (Jeno's), ½-oz. roll 2.5

pizza snacks:

    cheese (Jeno's Snack Tray), 1 pizza** 4.8

    pepperoni (Jeno's Snack Tray), 1 pizza** 4.7

    sausage (Jeno's Snack Tray), 1 pizza** 4.6

puff pastry hors d'oeuvres:

    beef (Durkee), ½-oz. puff 3.1

    cheese (Durkee), ½-oz. puff 2.9

    chicken (Durkee), ½-oz. puff 3.1

    chicken liver (Durkee), ½-oz. puff 3.1

    shrimp (Durkee), ½-oz. puff 3.0

snack logs:

    fish and chips (Jeno's), 2-oz. log 14.9

    Reuben (Jeno's), 2-oz. log 11.7

    sausage (Jeno's), 2-oz. log 12.5

tacos (Patio Cocktail), ½-oz. taco 4.9

* *Somewhat over one-quarter ounce*
** *Somewhat under one-half ounce*

APPETIZERS, HORS D'OEUVRES & SNACKS, CANNED, DRIED AND IN JARS

See also "Appetizers, Hors d'Oeuvres & Snacks, Frozen,"
"Meat, Fish & Poultry Spreads," "Fish & Seafood, Canned," etc.

GRAMS

anchovies, rolled, w/capers (Cresca), 2-oz. tin 9

caviar, in jars:

    black, sturgeon, whole grain (Northland Queen), 1 oz. 9

caviar, continued

black, sturgeon, whole grain (Romanoff—all seals), 1 oz. 1.1
chicken livers, chopped, canned (Reese), 1 oz. 9
franks, cocktail, in jars (Cresca), 1 oz. 0
franks, cocktail, vacuum sealed (Vienna), 1 oz. 7
gefilte fish, cocktail, in jars:
   (Manischewitz Fishlets), 1 piece 3
   whitefish-pike (Manischewitz Deluxe Fishlets), 1 piece 2
herring, kippered, canned (King Oscar Kipper Snacks), 3¼-oz. can ...0
meatballs, cocktail, canned (Cresca), 1 oz. 0
mussels, in natural juice, canned (Cresca), 1 oz. 9
pâté, canned:
   de foie gras*, 1 oz. 1.4
   (Cresca Pâté Au Foie), 1 oz. 1.3
   (Cresca Pâté Maison), 1 oz. 1.4
   (Cresca Smoked Goose Pâté) 1 oz. 3.1
   w/truffles (Le Parfait Swiss Pâté), 1 oz. 3.1
salami, Danish cocktail, canned (Cresca), 1 oz. ....tr.
salami sticks, Danish cocktail, canned (Cresca), 1 oz. ....tr.
salami sticks, Danish cocktail, canned (Reese), 1 oz. 3
sausage, cocktail, canned (Cresca), 1 oz. 0
sausage, dried, rolled:
   (Cow-Boy Jo's Beef Jerky), ¼-oz. pkg. 4
   (Cow-Boy Jo's Beef Sausage), ⅝-oz. pkg. 9
   (Cow-Boy Jo's Smok-O-Roni Beef Sausage), ¼-oz. pkg. 3
   (Lowrey's Pickled Hot Sausage), 1¼-oz. pkg. 1.4
   (Lowrey's Pickled Polish Sausage), ⅝-oz. pkg. 4
sausage, Vienna, canned:
   (Armour Star), 1 oz. ....tr.
   (Libby's), 1 oz. 1
   (Wilson's Certified), 1 oz. 1
shrimp, Danish cocktail, in jars (Cresca), 1 oz. 4

* *Data from United States Department of Agriculture*

CHAPTER 9

SOUPS, BROTHS AND CHOWDERS

SOUPS, BROTHS & CHOWDERS,
eight-ounce cup, except as noted

	GRAMS
alphabet, mix, prepared* (Golden Grain)	9.0
asparagus, cream of, cond., prepared* (Campbell's)	13.0
bean:	
cond., prepared* (Manischewitz)	17.6
w/bacon, cond., prepared* (Campbell's)	22.3
w/hot dogs, cond., prepared* (Campbell's Hot Dog Bean)	23.0
w/smoked ham, ready to serve (Great American)	24.5
w/smoked pork, cond., prepared* (Heinz)	20.1
bean, black, cond., prepared* (Campbell's)	14.4
bean, black, w/sherry, ready to serve (Crosse & Blackwell)	20.8
bean, lima, cond., prepared* (Manischewitz)	15.3
beef:	
cond., prepared* (Campbell's)	11.2
bouillon (Herb-Ox), 1 cube	.5
bouillon (Knorr Swiss), 1 cube	tr.
bouillon (Maggi), 1 cube or 1 tsp. mix	.5
bouillon (Wyler's), 1 cube or 1 tsp. mix	.5
broth, ready to serve (College Inn)	7.4
broth, ready to serve (Swanson)	.3

beef, continued

broth, cond., prepared* (Campbell's) 2.5
broth, mix (Maggi Broth & Seasoning), 1 tsp. 1.5
broth, mix (MBT), 1 packet 1
consommé, see "consommé, beef," page 82
barley, cond., prepared* (Manischewitz) 12.2
barley, mix, prepared* (Wyler's) 13.0
w/beef chunks and vegetables, ready to serve
  (Campbell's Chunky) 19.8
w/cabbage, cond., prepared* (Manischewitz) 9.8
noodle, cond., prepared* (Campbell's) 8.5
noodle, cond., prepared* (Heinz) 6.7
noodle, cond., prepared* (Manischewitz) 8.6
noodle, mix, prepared* (Lipton Cup-A-Soup), 6-oz. cup 6.3
noodle, mix, prepared* (Wyler's) 9.0
noodle and dumplings, ready to serve (Great American) 11.1
noodle, w/vegetables, mix, prepared* (Lipton) 11.0
w/vegetables, cond., prepared* (Manischewitz) 9.6
borscht, ready to serve (Manischewitz) 17.3
borscht, ready to serve (Mother's) 21.0
borscht, ready to serve (Rokeach) 17.8
celery, cream of, cond., prepared* (Campbell's) 7.6
celery, cream of, cond., prepared* (Heinz) 9.0
cheddar cheese, cond., prepared* (Campbell's) 10.4
chicken:
  bouillon (Herb-Ox), 1 cube 5
  bouillon (Knorr Swiss) ....tr.
  bouillon (Maggi), 1 cube or 1 tsp. mix 1.1
  bouillon (Wyler's), 1 cube or 1 tsp. mix ....tr.
  broth, ready to serve (College Inn) 1
  broth, ready to serve (Richardson & Robbins) 1.6
  broth, ready to serve (Swanson) 3
  broth, cond., prepared* (Campbell's) 1.4
  broth, mix (Maggi Broth & Seasoning), 1 tsp. 1.8
  broth, mix (MBT), 1 packet ....tr.
  broth, w/rice, ready to serve (Richardson & Robbins) 4.8
  barley, cond., prepared* (Manischewitz) 13.4

chicken, continued

w/chicken chunks and vegetables, ready to serve
(Campbell's Chunky) 16.7

consommé, see "consommé, chicken flavor," page 82

cream of, ready to serve (Great American) 9.0

cream of, cond., prepared* (Campbell's) 7.5

cream of, cond., prepared* (Heinz) 8.3

w/dumplings, cond., prepared* (Campbell's) 5.0

egg drop, cond., prepared* (Temple) 5.0

gumbo, cond., prepared* (Campbell's) 8.9

gumbo, creole style, ready to serve (Great American) 15.0

w/kasha, cond., prepared* (Manischewitz) 5.7

w/macaroni stars, cond., prepared* (Campbell's) 7.2

noodle, cond., prepared* (Campbell's) 8.4

noodle, cond., prepared* (Heinz) 9.5

noodle, cond., prepared* (Manischewitz) 4.4

noodle, mix, prepared* (Golden Grain) 8.8

noodle, mix, prepared* (Lipton Cup-A-Soup), 6-oz. cup 5.8

noodle, mix, prepared* (Wyler's) 5.0

noodle, w/diced chicken, mix, prepared* (Lipton) 8.9

noodle, w/dumplings, ready to serve (Great American) 8.9

w/noodle rings, cond., prepared* (Campbell's Noodle-O's) 9.3

w/noodle stars, cond., prepared* (Heinz) 7.9

rice, cond., prepared* (Campbell's) 5.8

rice, cond., prepared* (Heinz) 6.7

rice, cond., prepared* (Manischewitz) 5.8

rice, mix, prepared* (Golden Grain Chicken Rice-A-Roni) 10.9

rice, mix, prepared* (Lipton) 8.0

rice, mix, prepared* (Wyler's) 8.0

rice, w/mushrooms, ready to serve (Great American) 11.6

vegetable, cond., prepared* (Campbell's) 9.3

vegetable, cond., prepared* (Heinz) 9.3

vegetable, cond., prepared* (Manischewitz) 7.7

vegetable, mix, prepared* (Lipton) 10.2

vegetable, mix, prepared* (Wyler's) 5.0

chili beef, ready to serve (Great American) 22.0

chili beef, cond., prepared* (Campbell's) 22.8

Soups, Broths & Chowders, continued

chili beef, cond., prepared* (Heinz) 21.2
chowder:
    clam, Manhattan, ready to serve (Campbell's Chunky) 17.8
    clam, Manhattan, ready to serve (Crosse & Blackwell) 17.3
    clam, Manhattan, ready to serve (Great American) 14.2
    clam, Manhattan, cond., prepared* (Campbell's) 11.2
    clam, Manhattan, cond., prepared* (Snow's) 7.8
    clam, New England, ready to serve (Crosse & Blackwell) 13.8
    clam, New England, cond., prepared* (Campbell's) 16.9
    clam, New England, cond., prepared* (Snow's) 16.9
    corn, New England, cond., prepared* (Snow's) 20.0
    fish, New England, cond., prepared* (Snow's) 11.9
    sea food, New England, cond., prepared* (Snow's) 12.7
clam broth, mix (Maggi Broth & Seasoning), 1 tsp. 1.8
clam stew, cream of, cond., prepared* (Snow's) 12.9
consommé:
    beef, cond., prepared* (Campbell's) 3.0
    beef flavor, mix, prepared* (Knorr Swiss) 4
    chicken flavor, mix, prepared* (Knorr Swiss) 3
    Madrilene, clear, ready to serve (Crosse & Blackwell) 3.2
    Madrilene, red, ready to serve (Crosse & Blackwell) 3.2
    oxtail flavor, mix, prepared* (Knorr Swiss) 7
    w/noodles, mix, prepared* (Knorr Swiss Célestine) 7.2
crab, ready to serve (Crosse & Blackwell) 11.3
gazpacho, ready to serve (Crosse & Blackwell) 9.1
leek, mix, prepared* (Knorr Swiss) 10.3
lentil, ready to serve (La Rosa) 20.2
lentil, cond., prepared* (Manischewitz) 29.5
lentil, w/ham, ready to serve (Crosse & Blackwell) 20.5
lobster bisque, w/sherry, ready to serve (Crosse & Blackwell) 8.7
lobster, cream of, ready to serve (Crosse & Blackwell) 8.6
luk-shen, cond., prepared* (Temple) 8.0
minestrone:
    ready to serve (Crosse & Blackwell) 19.4
    ready to serve (La Rosa) 11.9

minestrone, continued

    cond., prepared* (Campbell's) 11.2

    mix, prepared* (Golden Grain) 11.2

mushroom:

    cond., prepared* (Campbell's) 8.2

    mix, prepared* (Golden Grain) 16.0

    w/barley, cond., prepared* (Manischewitz) 13.2

    w/beef flavor, mix, prepared* (Lipton) 6.2

    bisque, ready to serve (Crosse & Blackwell) 10.9

    cream of, ready to serve (Great American) 12.4

    cream of, cond., prepared* (Campbell's) 8.9

    cream of, cond., prepared* (Heinz) 10.4

noodle:

    w/chicken, cond., prepared* (Campbell's Curly Noodle) 9.9

    w/chicken flavor, mix, prepared* (Knorr Swiss) 10.1

    w/chicken broth, mix, prepared* (Lipton) 7.2

    w/chicken broth, mix, prepared* (Lipton Giggle Noodle) 11.3

    w/chicken broth, mix, prepared* (Lipton Ring-O) 9.4

    w/ground beef, cond., prepared* (Campbell's) 9.9

onion:

    ready to serve (Crosse & Blackwell) 6.3

    cond., prepared* (Campbell's) 3.2

    mix, prepared* (Golden Grain) 7.0

    mix, prepared* (Knorr Swiss) 7.6

    mix, prepared* (Lipton) 5.5

    mix, prepared* (Lipton Cup-A-Soup), 6-oz. cup 5.2

    bouillon, mix (Wyler's), 1 cube 1.0

    broth, mix (Maggi Broth & Seasoning), 1 tsp. 1.9

oxtail, mix, prepared* (Knorr Swiss) 8.3

oxtail, w/sherry, ready to serve (Crosse & Blackwell) 9.9

oyster stew, cond., prepared* (Campbell's) 12.1

pea, green:

    cond., prepared* (Campbell's) 23.6

    mix, prepared* (Golden Grain) 21.0

    mix, prepared* (Knorr Swiss) 8.4

    mix, prepared* (Lipton) 22.6

pea, green, continued

    mix, prepared* (Lipton Cup-A-Soup), 6-oz. cup 21.8

pea, split:

    cond., prepared* (Manischewitz) 22.5

    w/smoked ham, ready to serve (Great American) 24.0

    w/ham, cond., prepared* (Campbell's) 24.4

    w/ham, cond., prepared* (Heinz) 23.0

pepper pot, cond., prepared* (Campbell's) 9.5

Petite Marmite, ready to serve (Crosse & Blackwell) 5.0

potato, mix, prepared* (Lipton) 18.6

potato, cream of, cond., prepared* (Campbell's) 13.7

potato, cream of, w/leeks, mix, prepared* (Wyler's) 12.0

schav, ready to serve (Manischewitz) 2.0

Scotch broth, cond., prepared* (Campbell's) 10.5

Senegalese, ready to serve (Crosse & Blackwell) 9.1

shrimp, cream of, ready to serve (Crosse & Blackwell) 8.6

shrimp, cream of, cond., prepared* (Campbell's) 12.8

sirloin burger, ready to serve (Campbell's Chunky) 15.1

tomato:

    ready to serve (Great American) 26.3

    cond., prepared* (Campbell's) 15.0

    cond., prepared* (Heinz) 17.3

    cond., prepared* (Manischewitz) 9.6

    mix, prepared* (Lipton Cup-A-Soup), 6-oz. cup 17.3

    w/beef and noodles, cond., prepared*
      (Campbell's Tomato-Beef Noodle-O's) 17.0

    bisque, cond., prepared* (Campbell's) 23.0

    rice, cond., prepared* (Campbell's) 17.9

    rice, cond., prepared* (Manischewitz) 12.8

    vegetable, ready to serve (Great American) 17.6

    vegetable, mix, prepared* (Golden Grain) 13.3

    vegetable, w/noodles, mix, prepared* (Lipton) 11.7

tuna creole, ready to serve (Crosse & Blackwell) 8.8

turkey:

    noodle, ready to serve (Great American) 12.1

    noodle, cond., prepared* (Campbell's) 7.8

    noodle, cond., prepared* (Heinz) 10.0

turkey, continued

noodle, mix, prepared* (Lipton) 7.3

rice, w/mushrooms, ready to serve (Great American) 13.2

w/turkey chunks and vegetables, ready to serve
(Campbell's Chunky) 11.4

vegetable, ready to serve (Great American) 13.2

vegetable, cond., prepared* (Campbell's) 8.5

vegetable (see also "vegetarian vegetable," below):

cond., prepared* (Campbell's) 13.5

cond., prepared* (Campbell's Old Fashioned) 9.5

mix, prepared* (Wyler's) 9.0

bouillon (Herb-Ox), 1 cube 5

bouillon (Wyler's), 1 cube 5

broth, mix (Maggi Broth & Seasoning), 1 tsp. 1.5

broth, mix (MBT), 1 packet ....tr.

w/beef broth, ready to serve (Great American) 18.4

w/beef stock, ready to serve (Campbell's Chunky) 17.4

w/beef stock, cond., prepared* (Campbell's Stockpot) 9.1

w/beef stock, cond., prepared* (Heinz) 13.4

beef, ready to serve (Great American) 12.2

beef, cond., prepared* (Campbell's) 7.8

beef, cond., prepared* (Heinz) 9.6

beef, mix, prepared* (Lipton) 7.9

w/ground beef, ready to serve (Great American) 12.1

w/noodles, cond., prepared* (Campbell's Vegetable Noodle-O's) ..11.0

w/noodles, mix, prepared* (Lipton) 13.6

vegetarian vegetable:

ready to serve (Great American) 18.1

cond., prepared* (Campbell's) 12.7

cond., prepared* (Heinz) 14.2

cond., prepared* (Manischewitz) 10.1

mix, prepared* (Knorr Swiss) 5.5

vermicelli, w/meatballs, mix, prepared* (Knorr Swiss) 10.4

vichyssoise, ready to serve (Crosse & Blackwell) 12.4

won ton, cond., prepared* (Temple) 8.5

* *According to package directions*

CHAPTER 10

VEGETABLES, RELISHES AND VEGETABLE JUICES

VEGETABLES, FRESH*

See also "Vegetables, Canned, Frozen & Mixes"

GRAMS

artichoke, French, boiled or steamed, 1 large (about 7 oz.) 7.9
artichoke, Jerusalem, raw, pared, 4 oz. 18.9
asparagus, boiled, drained, 5-6 spears 3.5
asparagus, cut, boiled, drained, ½ cup 3.1
avocado, see "Fruits, Fresh," page 25
bamboo shoots, raw, ½ cup 3.9
bean sprouts:
   mung, raw, 4 oz. 7.5
   mung, boiled, drained, 4 oz. 5.9
   soy, raw, 4 oz. 6.0
   soy, boiled, drained, 4 oz. 4.2
beans, green or snap, raw, cut, ½ cup 3.6
beans, green or snap, whole, boiled, drained, 4 oz. 6.1
beans, green or snap, cut, boiled, drained, ½ cup 3.4
beans, kidney, red, boiled, drained, ½ cup 17.1
beans, kidney, white, boiled, drained, ½ cup 17.1
beans, lima, immature, boiled, drained, ½ cup 16.8
beans, lima, mature, boiled, drained, ½ cup 24.3
beans, wax or yellow, raw, cut, ½ cup 3.1

beans, wax or yellow, whole, boiled, drained, 4 oz. 5.2
beans, wax or yellow, cut, boiled, drained, ½ cup 3.7
beans, soy, see "soybeans," page 91
beets, raw, 1 average, 2" diameter 4.9
beets, diced, boiled, drained, ½ cup 6.5
beets, sliced, boiled, drained, ½ cup 7.3
beet greens, raw, ½ lb. 11.7
beet greens, boiled, drained, ½ cup 2.4
broccoli, raw, ½ lb. 10.4
broccoli spears, boiled, drained, 4 oz. 5.1
broccoli, cut, boiled, drained, ½ cup 3.3
Brussels sprouts, boiled, drained, ½ cup 4.2
cabbage, common varieties:
  white, raw, ½ lb. 9.7
  white, raw, shredded, ½ cup 5.7
  white, shredded, boiled, drained, ½ cup 3.7
  red, raw, ½ lb. 14.1
  red, raw, shredded, ½ cup 7.2
  savoy, raw, ½ lb. 9.4
cabbage, Chinese or celery, raw, ½ lb. 6.6
cabbage, Chinese or celery, raw, cut, ½ cup 1.5
cabbage, spoon, raw, ½ lb. 6.3
cabbage, spoon, boiled, drained, ½ cup 1.8
carrots:
  raw, pared, 1 average, 5½" x 1" 4.8
  raw, grated or shredded, ½ cup 5.3
  raw, sliced, ½ cup 6.0
  diced, boiled, drained, ½ cup 4.8
  sliced, boiled, drained, ½ cup 5.2
cauliflower, raw, flowerbuds, ½ lb. 11.8
cauliflower, boiled, drained, ½ cup 2.5
celeriac, raw, 4-6 roots 8.5
celery:
  raw, 1 outer stalk, 8" long 1.6
  raw, diced, ½ cup 2.0
  diced, boiled, drained, ½ cup 2.3

celery, continued

sliced, boiled, drained, ½ cup 2.6
chard, Swiss, raw, ½ lb. 9.6
chard, Swiss, boiled, drained, ½ cup 3.2
chicory, wiltproof, see "endive, French or Belgian," below
chicory greens, trimmed, ½ lb. 8.6
chives, raw, trimmed, 2 oz. 3.3
chives, raw, cut, 1 tbsp. 2.0
collards:
    raw, leaves only, ½ lb. 11.6
    raw, leaves and stems, ½ lb. 16.4
    boiled in small amount water, drained, ½ cup 5.1
    boiled in large amount water, drained, ½ cup 4.8
corn, on the cob, boiled, 1 ear, 5" x 1¾" 16.4
corn, kernels, boiled, drained, ½ cup 15.6
cowpeas, immature, boiled, drained, ½ cup 14.4
cowpeas, mature, boiled, drained, ½ cup 17.2
cress, garden, raw, trimmed, ½ lb. 12.4
cress, garden, boiled, drained, ½ cup 3.3
cress, water, see "watercress," page 92
cucumber, raw:
    unpared, 1 average, 7½" x 2" 6.9
    pared, 1 average, 7½" x 2" 6.6
    pared, 6 slices, 2" x ⅛" 1.6
    pared, diced, ½ cup 2.3
dandelion greens, raw, trimmed, ½ lb. 20.9
dandelion greens, boiled, drained, ½ cup 5.8
dock or sorrel, raw, ½ lb. 9.0
dock or sorrel, boiled, drained, ½ cup 3.9
eggplant, diced, boiled, drained, ½ cup 4.1
endive, curly, see "escarole," below
endive, French or Belgian, raw, trimmed, ½ lb. 6.5
endive, French or Belgian, raw, 10 small leaves 1.0
endive, French or Belgian, raw, cut, ½ cup 7
escarole, raw, ½ lb. 8.2
escarole, raw, 7 small leaves 8
escarole, raw, cut or shredded, ½ cup 1.5

fennel leaves, raw, trimmed, ½ lb. 10.8
garlic, raw, 1 average clove 6
horseradish, raw, pared, 1 oz. 5.6
kale:
  raw, leaves only, ½ lb. 13.1
  raw, leaves and stems, ½ lb. 10.0
  leaves only, boiled, drained, ½ cup 2.2
  leaves and stems, boiled, drained, ½ cup 3.3
kohlrabi, raw, diced, ½ cup 4.5
kohlrabi, boiled, drained, ½ cup 4.1
leeks, raw, 3 average 11.2
lentils, whole, boiled, drained, ½ cup 18.5
lettuce, raw:
  Boston or bibb, 1 head, 4″ diameter 5.5
  iceberg, 1 head, 4¾″ diameter 13.2
  iceberg, 3 average leaves 1.3
  iceberg, chopped, 1 cup 1.9
  looseleaf or salad bowl, 2 large leaves 1.8
  romaine or cos, 3 leaves, 8″ long 1.0
  romaine or cos, shredded, 1 cup 1.6
mushrooms, raw, 4 oz. 4.9
mushrooms, raw, trimmed, sliced, ½ cup 1.5
mustard greens, raw, ½ lb. 8.9
mustard greens, boiled, drained, ½ cup 4.4
mustard spinach, raw, ½ lb. 8.9
mustard spinach, boiled, drained, 4 oz. 3.2
New Zealand spinach, raw, ½ lb. 7.0
New Zealand spinach, boiled, drained, 4 oz. 2.4
okra:
  raw, whole, ½ lb. 14.8
  boiled, drained, 8 pods, 3″ long 5.1
  sliced, boiled, drained, ½ cup 4.8
onions:
  raw, 1 average, 2½″ diameter 9.6
  raw, sliced, ½ cup 4.9
  raw, chopped, 1 tbsp. 1.0

onions, continued

   boiled, drained, 1 cup 13.6

   cut, boiled, drained, 1 cup 11.8

onions, green:

   raw, ½ lb. 18.6

   raw, wo/tops, 6 small 5.3

   raw, sliced, ½ cup 5.1

   raw, tops only, 1 oz. 1.6

onions, Welsh, raw, ½ lb. 9.6

parsley, raw, ½ lb. 19.3

parsley, raw, chopped, 1 tbsp. 3

parsnips, raw, ½ lb. 33.8

parsnips, cut, boiled, drained, ½ cup 11.5

pea pods, Chinese, raw, ½ lb. 25.9

pea pods, Chinese, boiled, drained, 4 oz. 10.8

peas, blackeye, see "cowpeas," page 88

peas, green, raw, shelled, ½ cup 9.8

peas, green, boiled, drained, ½ cup 9.7

peas, split, cooked, ½ cup 16.6

pepper, chili, green, raw, ½ lb. 15.1

pepper, chili, red, pods w/seeds, raw, ½ lb. 39.4

pepper, chili, red, pods wo/seeds, raw, ½ lb. 26.2

pepper, sweet:

   green, raw, wo/seeds, 1 average (about 6 per lb.) 3.0

   green, raw, chopped, ½ cup 3.5

   green, raw, sliced, ½ cup 1.9

   green, boiled, drained, sliced, ½ cup 2.6

   red, raw, wo/seeds, 1 average (about 6 per lb.) 4.3

   red, raw, sliced, ½ cup 2.8

potatoes:

   baked w/skin, 1 average (about 3 per lb. raw) 20.9

   baked wo/skin, 1 average (about 3 per lb. raw) 17.0

   boiled w/skin, 1 average (about 3 per lb. raw) 23.3

   boiled wo/skin, 1 average (about 3 per lb. raw) 17.7

   French-fried in deep fat, 10 pieces, 2" x ½" x ½" 20.5

potatoes, sweet:

   baked w/skin, 1 average (about 6 oz. raw) 35.8

potatoes, sweet, continued

baked wo/skin, 1 average (about 6 oz. raw) 21.0
boiled w/skin, 1 average (about 6 oz. raw) 38.7
boiled wo/skin, 1 average (about 6 oz. raw) 31.3
pumpkin, raw, pulp only, 4 oz. 7.4
purslane leaves, raw, ½ lb. 8.6
purslane leaves, boiled, drained, ½ cup 2.5
radishes, raw, 4 small 1.4
radishes, raw, sliced, ½ cup 2.0
rutabagas, boiled, drained, ½ cup 8.2
scallions, see "onions, green," page 90
soybeans:
immature seeds, boiled, drained, 4 oz. 11.5
mature seeds, cooked, 4 oz. 12.2
sprouts, see "bean sprouts," page 86
curd, 4 oz. 2.7
spinach, raw, trimmed, ½ lb. 9.8
spinach, raw, chopped, ½ cup 2.2
spinach, boiled, drained, ½ cup 3.3
spinach, mustard, see "mustard spinach," page 89
spinach, New Zealand, see "New Zealand spinach," page 89
squash:
summer, scallop, cut, boiled, drained, ½ cup 4.0
summer, yellow, cut, boiled, drained, ½ cup 3.3
summer, zucchini, cut, boiled, drained, ½ cup 2.6
winter, acorn, baked, mashed, ½ cup 14.4
winter, butternut, baked, mashed, ½ cup 18.0
winter, hubbard, baked, mashed, ½ cup 12.0
tomato, green, raw, ½ lb. 10.6
tomato, ripe:
raw, 1 average (about 3 per lb.) 7.0
raw, peeled, 1 average (about 3 per lb.) 6.2
raw, sliced, ½ cup 4.3
boiled, w/liquid, ½ cup 6.7
turnip greens, raw, trimmed, ½ lb. 11.4
turnip greens, boiled, drained, ½ cup 2.6
turnips, wo/tops, raw, ½ lb. 12.9

Vegetables, Fresh, continued

turnips, diced, boiled, drained, ½ cup 3.8
water chestnuts, Chinese, raw, ½ lb. 33.2
water chestnuts, Chinese, peeled, 4 oz. 21.5
watercress, raw, ½ lb. 6.3
watercress, trimmed, ½ cup 5
yams, see "potatoes, sweet," pages 90-91
zucchini, see "squash, summer," page 91

* *Data from United States Department of Agriculture*

VEGETABLES, CANNED, FROZEN & MIXES,
half cup, except as noted

See also "Vegetables, Fresh"

	GRAMS
artichoke hearts, frozen (Birds Eye Deluxe), 5-6 hearts	4.8
asparagus, canned:	
drained (Del Monte)	3.0
drained (Musselman's)	2.8
spears (Green Giant), 6 spears	1.7
cut tips, w/liquid (Stokely-Van Camp)	2.9
cuts, drained (Stokely-Van Camp)	3.3
cuts, w/liquid (Green Giant)	1.8
asparagus, frozen:	
spears (Birds Eye 5-Minute), ⅓ pkg.*	3.6
spears (Seabrook Farms), 6 spears	1.8
cuts (Birds Eye 5-Minute)	3.3
cuts and tips (Seabrook Farms)	2.5
spears, in Hollandaise sauce (Birds Eye), ⅓ pkg.*	3.2
cuts, in butter sauce (Green Giant), ⅓ pkg.*	2.6
cuts and tips, in Hollandaise sauce (Seabrook Farms)	5.0
bamboo shoots, canned (Chun King)	1.2
bamboo shoots, canned (La Choy)	1.0
bean sprouts, canned:	
(China Beauty)	1.6

bean sprouts, canned, continued

  (Chun King) 1.3
  (La Choy) 1.0
  (Mow Sang) 3.0
beans, baked, canned:
  pea beans (B & M) 25.6
  pea beans (Homemaker's) 24.4
  red kidney beans (B & M) 24.8
  red kidney beans (Homemaker's) 25.6
  yellow eye beans (B & M) 25.2
beans, baked-style, canned:
  in barbecue sauce (Campbell's Barbecue Beans) 30.6
  in molasses sauce (Heinz) 26.4
  in molasses and brown sugar sauce (Campbell's Old Fashioned)..24.1
  in tomato sauce (Heinz Vegetarian) 24.5
  smoke flavor, in tomato sauce (Heinz Campside) 25.6
  w/beef, in tomato sauce (Campbell's Beans 'n Beef) 19.9
  w/frankfurters, in tomato sauce
    (Heinz Minute Meal), 8¾-oz. can 38.0
  w/frankfurters, in tomato sauce
    (Hormel Mini-Meal), 7½-oz. can 28.9
  w/frankfurters, in tomato sauce (Van Camp's Beenee Weenee) ..27.8
  w/frankfurters, in tomato and molasses sauce (Campbell's) 17.8
  w/pork, in molasses sauce (Heinz Boston Style) 25.4
  w/pork, in tomato sauce (Campbell's) 24.4
  w/pork, in tomato sauce (Campbell's Home Style) 24.4
  w/pork, in tomato sauce (Heinz Pork 'N' Beans) 24.3
  w/pork, in tomato sauce (Van Camp's) 31.8
beans, butter, see "butterbeans," page 96
beans, chili, canned (Austex) 9.4
beans, chili, Mexican style, canned (Gebhardt), 4 oz. 59.0
beans, green or snap, canned:
  whole, drained (Comstock) 2.9
  whole, drained (Del Monte) 2.8
  whole, w/liquid (Green Giant) 2.3
  whole, w/liquid (Stokely-Van Camp) 4.4
  cut, drained (Comstock) 2.5

beans, green or snap, canned, continued

cut, drained (Del Monte) 2.8
cut, drained (Lord Mott's) 3.0
cut, w/liquid (Green Giant) 2.8
cut, w/liquid (Stokely-Van Camp) 4.4
French-style, drained (Comstock) 3.6
French-style, drained (Del Monte) 2.8
French-style, drained (Lord Mott's) 3.0
French-style, w/liquid (Green Giant) 2.8
French-style, w/liquid (Stokely-Van Camp) 4.3
Italian-style, drained (Del Monte) 4.7
seasoned, drained (Del Monte) 2.6

beans, green or snap, frozen:

whole (Birds Eye Deluxe), ⅓ pkg.* 5.2
cut (Birds Eye 5-Minute), ⅓ pkg.* 5.1
cut (Green Giant), ⅓ pkg.* 4.2
cut (Seabrook Farms) 4.0
French-style (Birds Eye 5-Minute), ⅓ pkg.* 5.1
French-style (Seabrook Farms) 4.5
Italian-style (Birds Eye 5-Minute), ⅓ pkg.* 4.1
cut, in butter sauce (Green Giant), ⅓ pkg.* 3.1
cut, in mushroom sauce (Seabrook Farms) 4.5
cut, w/mushrooms (Green Giant), ⅓ pkg.* 3.9
French-style, in butter sauce (Green Giant), ⅓ pkg.* 2.6
French-style, w/almonds (Birds Eye) 6.0
French-style, w/sautéed mushrooms (Birds Eye), ⅓ pkg.* ...5.5
and spaetzle, in sauce (Birds Eye Bavarian-style), ⅓ pkg.* ...11.8

beans, kidney, dark, canned, w/liquid (Van Camp's) 23.6
beans, kidney, light, canned, w/liquid (Van Camp's) 23.6
beans, kidney, red, canned, w/liquid
(Van Camp's New Orleans-Style) 27.2

beans, lima, canned:

drained (Del Monte) 17.0
green, all sizes, w/liquid (Stokely-Van Camp) 21.3
seasoned, drained (Del Monte) 15.9

beans, lima, frozen:

baby (Birds Eye 5-Minute) 21.0

beans, lima, frozen, continued

baby (Green Giant), ⅓ pkg.* 18.6
baby (Seabrook Farms) 16.0
Fordhook (Birds Eye 5-Minute), ⅓ pkg.* 17.9
Fordhook (Seabrook Farms) 16.0
baby, in butter sauce (Green Giant), ⅓ pkg.* 15.6
Fordhook, in cheese sauce (Seabrook Farms) 23.5
beans, mixed, in oil and vinegar, canned, w/liquid
(Green Giant 3-Bean Salad) 12.6
beans, October, canned, w/liquid (Van Camp's) 24.2
beans, pinto, canned (Old El Paso) 23.6
beans, pinto, w/chili, canned (Old El Paso Mexe Beans) 24.6
beans, refried, canned (Old El Paso) 23.0

beans, wax or yellow:

whole, canned, drained (Del Monte) 2.5
whole, canned, w/liquid (Stokely-Van Camp) 4.7
cut, canned, drained (Comstock) 2.9
cut, canned, drained (Del Monte) 2.5
cut, canned w/liquid (Stokely-Van Camp) 4.7
cut, frozen (Birds Eye 5-Minute), ⅓ pkg.* 5.4
cut, frozen (Seabrook Farms) 4.0
French-style, canned, w/liquid (Stokely-Van Camp) 4.7

beets:

whole, all sizes, canned, w/liquid (Stokely-Van Camp) 9.0
whole, canned, drained (Del Monte) 6.1
diced, canned, w/liquid (Stokely-Van Camp) 9.1
sliced, canned, drained (Comstock) 6.2
sliced, canned, drained (Del Monte) 6.1
sliced, canned, drained (Lord Mott's) 6.2
sliced, canned, w/liquid (Stokely-Van Camp) 9.1
Harvard, canned, w/liquid (Greenwood) 12.9
Harvard, canned, w/liquid (Lord Mott's) 10.0
Harvard, canned, w/liquid (Stokely-Van Camp) 14.0
pickled, canned, drained (Del Monte Crinkle Cut) 14.8
pickled, canned, drained (Greenwood) 15.1
pickled, canned, w/liquid (Lord Mott's) 23.8
pickled, canned, w/liquid (Stokely-Van Camp) 19.6

beets, continued

in orange flavor glaze, frozen (Birds Eye), ⅓ pkg.* 14.9
broccoli, frozen:
   spears, baby (Birds Eye Deluxe), ⅓ pkg.* 3.6
   spears (Birds Eye 5-Minute), ⅓ pkg.* 3.6
   spears (Green Giant), ⅓ pkg.* 3.3
   spears (Seabrook Farms) 3.5
   chopped (Birds Eye 5-Minute), ⅓ pkg.* 3.6
   chopped (Seabrook Farms) 4.0
   spears, in butter sauce (Green Giant), ⅓ pkg.* 4.3
   spears, in Hollandaise sauce (Birds Eye), ⅓ pkg.* 3.2
   cuts, in cheese sauce (Green Giant), ⅓ pkg.* 5.6
   and noodles, in sour cream sauce
     (Green Giant Casserole), ⅓ pkg.* 9.6
Brussels sprouts, frozen:
   (Green Giant), ⅓ pkg.* 6.1
   (Seabrook Farms) 6.0
   baby (Birds Eye Deluxe) 5.7
   au gratin (Green Giant Casserole), ⅓ pkg.* 8.3
   in butter sauce (Green Giant), ⅓ pkg.* 4.7
butterbeans, canned, w/liquid (Stokely-Van Camp) 25.4
butterbeans, frozen (Birds Eye), ⅓ pkg.* 23.6
butterbeans, frozen (Seabrook Farms) 19.5
cabbage, canned:
   red, sweet and sour, w/liquid (Greenwood) 18.1
   red, sweet and sour, w/liquid (Lord Mott's) 15.0
   sauerkraut, w/liquid (Del Monte) 3.8
   sauerkraut, chopped, w/liquid (Stokely-Van Camp) 4.4
   sauerkraut, shredded, w/liquid (Stokely-Van Camp) 4.4
   sauerkraut, w/caraway, w/liquid
     (Stokely-Van Camp Bavarian-Style) 5.3
carrots:
   cut, canned, drained (Comstock) 5.7
   cut, canned, drained (Del Monte) 5.0
   cut, canned, drained (Lord Mott's) 5.0
   cut, canned, w/liquid (Stokely-Van Camp) 6.0
   nuggets, frozen (Green Giant), ⅓ pkg.* 7.1

carrots, continued

nuggets, in butter sauce, frozen (Green Giant), ⅓ pkg.* 6.0
nuggets, w/brown sugar glaze, frozen (Birds Eye) 16.8
sliced, w/honey glaze, frozen (Green Giant), ⅓ pkg.* 12.6
and peas, see "peas and carrots," page 100
cauliflower, frozen:
(Birds Eye 5-Minute), ⅓ pkg.* 3.2
(Seabrook Farms) 3.5
au gratin (Stouffer's), 10-oz. pkg. 17.9
in butter sauce (Green Giant), ⅓ pkg.* 3.3
in cheese sauce (Green Giant), ⅓ pkg.* 5.6
in sour cream sauce
(Green Giant Hungarian Casserole), ⅓ pkg.* 7.7
sweet, see "Olives, Pickles & Other Relishes," page 104
chick peas, see "garbanzos," page 98
collard greens, chopped, frozen (Birds Eye) ⅓ pkg.* 4.5
collard greens, chopped, frozen (Seabrook Farms) 4.0
corn, golden, canned:
on the cob (Stokely-Van Camp), 1 ear 17.0
drained (Del Monte) 16.4
w/liquid (Green Giant) 18.4
w/liquid (Stokely-Van Camp) 19.0
vacuum-pack, w/liquid (Del Monte) 19.6
vacuum-pack, w/liquid (Green Giant) 19.1
vacuum-pack, w/liquid (Stokely-Van Camp) 23.5
cream-style (Del Monte) 25.0
cream-style (Green Giant) 21.6
cream-style (Stokely-Van Camp) 23.7
and lima beans, see "succotash," page 102
w/peppers, w/liquid (Del Monte) 19.3
w/peppers, w/liquid (Green Giant Mexicorn) 18.8
corn, golden, frozen:
on the cob (Birds Eye), 1 ear 21.7
on the cob (Ore-Ida), 6" ear 28.0
(Birds Eye 5-Minute) 17.8
(Green Giant), ⅓ pkg.* 13.3
(Ore-Ida) 15.8

corn, golden, frozen, continued

   (Seabrook Farms) 16.5

   in butter sauce (Green Giant), ⅓ pkg.* 14.2

   in cheese sauce (Green Giant Swiss Casserole), ⅓ pkg.* 17.8

   w/peppers, in butter sauce (Green Giant Mexicorn), ⅓ pkg.* 14.3

   and lima beans, see "succotash," page 102

   and peas, w/tomatoes (Birds Eye), ⅓ pkg.* 15.0

corn, white:

   canned, w/liquid (Stokely-Van Camp) 19.0

   in butter sauce, frozen (Green Giant), ⅓ pkg.* 15.2

   w/peppers, in butter sauce, frozen
   (Green Giant Mexicorn), ⅓ pkg.* 19.5

eggplant Parmesan, frozen (Mrs. Paul's), 11-oz. pkg. 47.6

eggplant sticks, breaded, fried, frozen (Mrs. Paul's), 7-oz. pkg. 57.7

garbanzos, canned (Old El Paso) 16.7

hominy, golden or white, canned (Van Camp's) 15.0

kale, leaf, frozen (Seabrook Farms) 5.0

kale, chopped, frozen (Birds Eye) 4.2

kale, chopped, frozen (Seabrook Farms) 5.0

mushrooms:

   whole, canned, drained (Brandywine) 4.5

   whole, canned, w/liquid (Green Giant) 3.9

   sliced, canned, drained (Brandywine) 4.5

   sliced, canned, w/liquid (Green Giant) 3.3

   stems and pieces, canned, drained (Brandywine) 4.5

   stems and pieces, canned, w/liquid (Green Giant) 2.7

   in butter, canned (B in B) 4.5

   in butter sauce, frozen (Green Giant), 6-oz. pkg. 5.1

   pickled, see "Olives, Pickles & Other Relishes," page 104

mustard greens, leaf, frozen (Seabrook Farms) 3.5

mustard greens, chopped, frozen (Birds Eye) 2.2

mustard greens, chopped, frozen (Seabrook Farms) 3.5

okra, frozen:

   whole (Birds Eye) 5.7

   whole (Seabrook Farms) 6.0

   cut (Birds Eye) 7.6

   cut (Seabrook Farms) 6.0

onions, canned:

    whole, boiled (O & C) 7.8

    whole, boiled (Lord Mott's) 5.0

    in cream sauce (O & C) 9.2

    in cream-style sauce (Lord Mott's) 13.0

    French-fried rings (O & C), 3-oz. can 38.2

    pickled, see "Olives, Pickles & Other Relishes," page 104

onions, frozen:

    whole, small (Birds Eye) 12.0

    chopped (Birds Eye), ¼ cup 2.5

    chopped (Ore-Ida), ¼ cup 2.1

    in cream sauce (Birds Eye), ⅓ pkg.* 12.7

    in cream sauce (Green Giant), ⅓ pkg.* 6.6

    in cream sauce (Seabrook Farms) 5.5

    French-fried rings (Birds Eye), 4-oz. pkg. 34.2

    French-fried rings (Mrs. Paul's), 5-oz. pkg. 28.2

    French-fried rings (Ore-Ida), 4 average rings 18.0

peas, green, canned:

    early, w/liquid (Le Sueur) 9.1

    early, w/liquid (Stokely-Van Camp) 14.1

    sweet, drained (Comstock) 6.8

    sweet, drained (Del Monte) 7.3

    sweet, w/liquid (Green Giant) 8.3

    sweet, w/liquid (Stokely-Van Camp) 9.1

    seasoned, drained (Del Monte) 8.7

peas, green, frozen:

    early (Birds Eye Deluxe) 12.0

    early (Seabrook Farms) 12.5

    sweet (Birds Eye 5-Minute) 12.2

    sweet (Green Giant), ⅓ pkg.* 10.4

    sweet (Seabrook Farms) 9.0

    early, in butter sauce (Le Sueur), ⅓ pkg.* 9.6

    sweet, in butter sauce (Green Giant), ⅓ pkg.* 8.8

    in cream sauce (Birds Eye), ⅓ pkg.* 13.6

    in cream sauce (Green Giant), ⅓ pkg.* 9.3

    in onion sauce (Seabrook Farms) 10.0

peas, green, frozen, continued

w/celery (Birds Eye) 9.8
w/mushrooms (Birds Eye), ⅓ pkg.* 11.7
w/onions (Birds Eye), ⅓ pkg.* 12.3
w/onions, in butter sauce (Green Giant), ⅓ pkg.* 7.9
w/potatoes, in cream sauce (Birds Eye), ⅓ pkg.* 14.9
and rice, w/mushrooms (Birds Eye), ⅓ pkg.* 21.9

peas and carrots:
canned, drained (Del Monte) 6.8
canned, w/liquid (Lord Mott's) 10.5
canned, w/liquid (Stokely-Van Camp) 10.1
frozen (Birds Eye 5-Minute) 8.7
frozen (Seabrook Farms) 7.5
in butter sauce, frozen (Green Giant), ⅓ pkg.* 8.1

peppers, chili, see "Olives, Pickles & Other Relishes," page 105
pimientos, see "Olives, Pickles & Other Relishes," page 106

potatoes, canned:
new, whole, drained (Del Monte) 9.5
boiled (Lord Mott's) 11.1
boiled (Stokely-Van Camp) 12.0
scalloped, w/ham (Hormel Mini-Meal), 7½-oz. can 17.0
sweet, see "potatoes, sweet," page 101

potatoes, frozen:
boiled (Seabrook Farms) 16.5
boiled, buttered, w/parsley (Seabrook Farms) 14.5
au gratin (Stouffer's), 11½-oz. pkg. 34.6
baked, stuffed, w/cheese topping (Holloway House), 12-oz. pkg. ..56.1
baked, stuffed, w/sour cream (Holloway House), 12-oz. pkg. 54.7
French-fried (Ore-Ida Cottage Fries), 17 pieces 19.7
French-fried (Ore-Ida Golden Crinkles), 17 pieces 16.3
French-fried (Ore-Ida Golden Fries), 17 pieces 15.5
French-fried (Ore-Ida Shoestrings), 25 pieces 9.0
French-fried (Seabrook Farms), 17 pieces 19.0
French-fried, bite-size (Ore-Ida Tater-Tots), 10 pieces 23.2
hash-brown, shredded (Ore-Ida) 13.2
sweet, see "potatoes, sweet," page 101

Vegetables, Canned, Frozen & Mixes, continued

potatoes, mixes, prepared**:
  au gratin (Betty Crocker) 20.8
  au gratin (French's) 16.0
  mashed (Betty Crocker Potato Buds) 17.1
  mashed (French's Country Style Flakes) 17.0
  mashed (Ore-Ida Potato Flakes) 22.2
  mashed (Pillsbury) 17.4
  pancakes (French's), 3 small 16.0
  scalloped (Betty Crocker) 22.2
  scalloped (French's) 20.0
  whipped (Borden's) 16.0
potatoes, sweet:
  canned, w/syrup (Green Giant) 23.6
  candied, frozen (Birds Eye), ⅓ pkg.* 53.3
  candied, frozen (Mrs. Paul's), ⅓ pkg. 45.0
  w/brown sugar pineapple glaze, frozen (Birds Eye) 30.7
pumpkin, canned (Del Monte) 9.6
pumpkin, canned (Stokely-Van Camp) 8.1
sauerkraut, see "cabbage," page 96
spinach, canned:
  drained (Del Monte) 3.0
  leaf, w/liquid (Stokely-Van Camp) 3.2
  leaf, w/liquid (Lord Mott's) 3.2
  chopped, w/liquid (Lord Mott's) 3.2
  chopped, w/liquid (Stokely-Van Camp) 3.2
  chopped, in cream-style sauce (Lord Mott's) 9.7
spinach, frozen:
  leaf (Birds Eye 5-Minute), ⅓ pkg.* 3.1
  leaf (Seabrook Farms) 4.0
  chopped (Birds Eye 5-Minute), ⅓ pkg.* 2.7
  chopped (Seabrook Farms) 4.0
  leaf, in butter sauce (Green Giant), ⅓ pkg.* 3.1
  leaf, in cream sauce (Green Giant), ⅓ pkg.* 4.3
  chopped, in butter sauce (Birds Eye) 3.0
  creamed (Birds Eye), ⅓ pkg.* 5.4

spinach, frozen, continued

    creamed (Seabrook Farms) 6.5
    deviled au gratin (Green Giant Casserole), ⅓ pkg.* 5.0
    soufflé (Stouffer's), 12-oz. pkg. 29.6
    soufflé (Swanson), 7½-oz. pkg. 15.9
squash:
    cooked, frozen (Birds Eye), ⅓ pkg.* 9.1
    cooked, frozen (Seabrook Farms) 11.0
    summer, sliced, frozen (Birds Eye 5-Minute) 3.8
    zucchini, frozen (Birds Eye), ⅓ pkg.* 2.3
    zucchini, breaded, fried, frozen (Mrs. Paul's), 9-oz. pkg. 63.0
    zucchini Parmesan, frozen (Mrs. Paul's), 12-oz. pkg. 16.1
    zucchini, in tomato sauce, canned (Del Monte) 5.6
succotash:
    canned, w/liquid (Stokely-Van Camp) 19.5
    frozen (Birds Eye 5-Minute) 19.4
    frozen (Seabrook Farms) 19.5
    cream-style, canned (Stokely-Van Camp) 20.0
tomato paste, see "Tomato Paste & Purée," page 107
tomato purée, see "Tomato Paste & Purée," page 107
tomatoes, canned:
    whole, w/liquid (Contadina) 3.5
    whole, w/liquid (Del Monte) 5.0
    whole, w/liquid (Hunt's) 5.1
    whole, w/liquid (Lord Mott's) 5.0
    whole, w/liquid (Stokely-Van Camp) 4.3
    wedges, w/liquid (Del Monte) 6.3
    sliced, baby, w/liquid (Contadina) 5.3
    sliced, w/liquid (Hunt's Italian-Style) 5.1
    stewed (Del Monte) 6.8
    stewed (Hunt's) 8.5
    stewed (Lord Mott's) 5.0
turnip greens:
    leaf, canned, w/liquid (Stokely-Van Camp) 3.6
    leaf, frozen (Seabrook Farms) 3.5
    chopped, canned, w/liquid (Stokely-Van Camp) 3.6
    chopped, frozen (Birds Eye) 2.7

turnip greens, continued
chopped, frozen (Seabrook Farms) 3.5
vegetables, mixed, canned:
  drained (Del Monte) 7.1
  w/liquid (Stokely-Van Camp) 13.4
  Chinese, see "Chinese Entrees & Side Dishes," page 131
  in oil and vinegar (Stokely-Van Camp SALADettes) 12.6
vegetables, mixed, frozen:
  (Birds Eye 5-Minute) 12.4
  (Seabrook Farms) 10.5
  in butter sauce (Green Giant), ⅓ pkg.* 8.3
  in cream sauce (Birds Eye Vegetable Jubilee) 18.7
  in onion sauce (Birds Eye) 13.6
  Chinese-style, in sauce (Birds Eye), ⅓ pkg.* 6.0
  Danish-style, in sauce (Birds Eye), ⅓ pkg.* 7.6
  Hawaiian-style, in sauce (Birds Eye), ⅓ pkg.* 12.6
  Italian-style, in sauce (Birds Eye), ⅓ pkg.* 7.9
  Japanese-style, in sauce (Birds Eye), ⅓ pkg.* 5.8
  Mexican-style, in sauce (Birds Eye), ⅓ pkg.* 17.0
  Parisian-style, in sauce (Birds Eye), ⅓ pkg.* 7.4
  Spanish-style, in sauce (Birds Eye Medley), ⅓ pkg.* 7.1
water chestnuts, canned (Chun King) 7.5
water chestnuts, canned (Lord Mott's), 5 pieces 7.8
yams, see "potatoes, sweet," page 101
zucchini, see "squash," page 102

  * *Approximately one-half cup, or slightly less*
 ** *According to package directions*

VEGETABLE JUICES, six-ounce glass, except as noted

	GRAMS
sauerkraut, canned*	4.3
tomato:	
bottled or canned (BC)	7.7
bottled (Welch's)	7.6

tomato juice, continued

canned (Campbell's) 6.6
canned (Del Monte) 7.4
canned (Hunt's) 7.8
canned (Libby's) 8.4
canned (Sacramento) 7.9
canned (Stokely-Van Camp) 8.5
dairy-pack (Sealtest), 4-oz. container 4.5
tomato cocktail, bottled or canned (Mott's) 9.0
tomato-beef broth cocktail, bottled or canned (Beefamato) 13.7
tomato-clam broth cocktail, bottled or canned (Clamato) 16.0
vegetable cocktail (V-8) 6.0

* *Data from United States Department of Agriculture*

OLIVES, PICKLES & OTHER RELISHES

	GRAMS

cauliflower, sweet (Smucker's), 1 bud 2.8
mushrooms, cocktail (Cresca), 3-oz. can* 2.8
mushrooms, cocktail (Reese Button), 4-oz. can* 3.7
olives:
   green, Manzanilla (Durkee), 1 medium ....tr.
   green, Manzanilla (Grandee), 1 medium ....tr.
   green, Spanish (Mario's), 1 medium 1
   green, pimiento-stuffed Manzanilla (Durkee), 1 queen size 2
   green, pimiento-stuffed Manzanilla (Grandee), 1 queen size 2
   green, salad, w/pimiento (Durkee), 1 tbsp. 3
   ripe (Durkee), 1 large 1
   ripe (Grandee), 1 large 1
   ripe (Lindsay), 1 large or extra large 1
   ripe (Lindsay), 1 giant or jumbo 2
   ripe (Lindsay), 1 colossal, super-colossal or super-supreme 3
onions, cocktail (Cresca), 1 onion ....tr.
onions, cocktail (Crosse & Blackwell), 1 tbsp. 3

peppers, hot:
  whole green chili (Cresca), 1 pepper 1
  whole green chili (Del Monte), 1 cup* 8.2
  whole green chili (Old El Paso), 4-oz. can* 5.6
  roasted, peeled, chopped chili (Old El Paso), 4-oz. can* 7.2
  whole, jalapeno (Old El Paso), 10-oz. can* 20.0
peppers, mild, sweet (Del Monte), 1 cup* 9.1
pickle and other relishes, one tablespoon:
  barbecue (Crosse & Blackwell) 5.4
  barbecue (Heinz) 8.5
  corn (Crosse & Blackwell) 3.6
  hamburger (Crosse & Blackwell) 4.7
  hamburger (Del Monte) 8.8
  hamburger (Heinz) 3.6
  hot dog (Crosse & Blackwell) 5.4
  hot dog (Del Monte) 6.7
  hot dog (Heinz) 3.9
  hot pepper (Crosse & Blackwell) 5.4
  India (Crosse & Blackwell) 6.3
  India (Heinz) 3.9
  mustard (Crosse & Blackwell Chow Chow) 9
  onion, spicy (Crosse & Blackwell) 4.2
  piccalilli (Crosse & Blackwell) 6.3
  piccalilli, green tomato (Heinz) 5.3
  picnic, tangy (Crosse & Blackwell) 5.0
  sweet (Crosse & Blackwell) 6.3
  sweet (Del Monte) 9.3
  sweet (Heinz) 6.6
  sweet (L & S) 4.0
  sweet (Smucker's) 5.0
pickles, dill:
  whole (Bond's Flavor-Pack), 1 average pickle 2
  whole (Bond's Fresh-Pack Kosher), 1 average pickle 2
  whole (Del Monte), 1 large pickle 1.4
  whole (Heinz Genuine), 4"-long pickle 1.1
  whole (Heinz Processed), 3"-long pickle 1

pickles, dill, continued

whole (L & S), 1 large pickle 2.0
whole (L & S Fresh-Pack Kosher), 1 large pickle 2.0
whole (Smucker's), 1 average pickle 1.3
whole (Smucker's Fresh-Pack Kosher), 1 average pickle 1.3
whole (Smucker's Kosher Baby), 1 average pickle 1.0
sticks (Smucker's Fresh-Pack Kosher), 1 large stick 1.0
spears (Bond's Fresh-Pack), 1 large spear 2
spears (Bond's Fresh-Pack Kosher), 1 large spear 2
slices (Crosse & Blackwell), 1 tbsp. 2.0
slices (Heinz Hamburger), 3 slices 1
slices (Smucker's Hamburger), 3 slices 5

pickles, sweet:

whole (Bond's Gherkins), 1 average pickle 3.0
whole (Heinz Gherkins), 2"-long pickle 3.9
whole (L & S), 1 large pickle 7.0
whole (Smucker's), 1 large pickle 6.3
whole (Smucker's Candied Midgets), 1 average pickle 2.5
whole (Smucker's Mixed), 1 average pickle 5.8
sticks (Smucker's Candied Dill), 1 large stick 9.0
sticks (Smucker's Fresh-Pack), 1 average stick 4.0
spears (Crosse & Blackwell Fresh Cucumber), 1 large spear 7.2
slices (Bond's Fresh-Pack Cucumber), 3 slices 5.0
slices (Crosse & Blackwell Fresh Cucumber), 1 tbsp. 3.7
slices (Fanning's Bread and Butter), 3 slices 3.6
slices (Heinz Cucumber), 3 slices 4.7
slices (L & S), 3 slices 4.0
pieces (Crosse & Blackwell Mixed), 1 tbsp. 4.9
pieces (Heinz Mixed), 3 pieces 5.6
chips (Crosse & Blackwell), 1 tbsp. 4.2
chips (Smucker's), 3 chips 6.0
chips (Smucker's Fresh-Pack), 3 chips 5.3

pimientos (Dromedary), 4 oz.* 4.7
pimientos (Stokely-Van Camp), ½ cup* 6.4
watermelon rind (Crosse & Blackwell), 1 tbsp. 9.3

* *Drained of liquid*

TOMATO PASTE & PURÉE, half cup, except as noted

	GRAMS
paste (Contadina), 6-oz. can	35.4
paste (Del Monte)	25.1
paste (Hunt's)	24.5
purée (Contadina)	9.1
purée (Hunt's)	10.5
purée (Lord Mott's)	10.1

CHAPTER 11

FROZEN DINNERS
AND POT PIES

FROZEN DINNERS, one complete dinner*

	GRAMS
beef:	
(Banquet), 11 oz.	20.2
(Freezer Queen Mini Meal), 6 oz.	11.5
(Morton), 11 oz.	22.0
(Morton—3-course), 17 oz.	60.1
(Swanson TV), 11½ oz.	30.3
(Swanson TV—3-course), 15 oz.	57.8
beef, chopped (Banquet), 9 oz.	26.9
beef, chopped (Swanson TV), 10 oz.	40.0
beef patty, char-broiled (Freezer Queen Mini Meal), 7½ oz.	15.1
catfish (Taste O'Sea), 9 oz.	37.5
chicken:	
(Banquet), 11 oz.	48.2
(Morton), 11 oz.	37.2
(Morton—3-course), 17 oz.	73.2
(Swanson TV), 11½ oz.	46.6
(Swanson TV—3-course), 15 oz.	62.6
(Swanson Hungry Man), 19 oz.	63.7
chicken croquette (Freezer Queen Mini Meal), 6½ oz.	23.0
chicken and dumplings (Morton), 12 oz.	30.7
chicken and dumplings (Morton—3-course), 16½ oz.	90.7

Frozen Dinners, continued

Chinese (Swanson TV International), 11 oz. 40.9
Chinese (Temple), 12 oz. 53.0
chop suey, beef (Banquet), 11 oz. 35.0
chow mein:
   beef (Chun King), 11 oz. 47.9
   chicken (Banquet), 11 oz. 32.0
   chicken (Chun King), 11 oz. 39.9
   shrimp (Chun King), 11 oz. 44.9
egg foo young (Chun King), 11 oz. 45.3
enchilada:
   beef (Banquet), 12½ oz. 61.1
   beef (Patio), 12 oz. 87.5
   beef (Swanson TV International), 15 oz. 59.5
   cheese (Banquet), 12½ oz. 58.3
   cheese (Patio), 12 oz. 88.0
fish (see also individual fish listings):
   (Morton), 8¾ oz. 42.4
   (Taste O'Sea), 9 oz. 43.6
   ocean, fillet of (Swanson TV), 12¼ oz. 36.5
fish cake (Taste O'Sea), 8 oz. 45.8
flounder (Taste O'Sea), 9 oz. 34.2
franks and beans (Banquet), 10¾ oz. 61.7
franks and beans (Morton), 12 oz. 81.3
franks and beans (Swanson TV), 11½ oz. 65.7
German (Swanson TV International), 11 oz. 42.2
haddock (Banquet), 8.8 oz. 44.6
haddock (Taste O'Sea), 9 oz. 35.5
ham (Banquet), 10 oz. 53.2
ham (Morton), 10 oz. 49.1
ham (Swanson TV), 10¼ oz. 42.1
Italian (Banquet), 11 oz. 44.0
Italian (Swanson TV International), 13½ oz. 54.1
macaroni and beef (Morton), 11 oz. 56.3
macaroni and beef (Swanson TV), 11.3 oz. 35.0
macaroni and cheese (Banquet), 12 oz. 47.0
macaroni and cheese (Morton), 12¾ oz. 38.5

Frozen Dinners, continued

macaroni and cheese (Swanson TV), 11.3 oz. 46.9
meatballs, w/gravy (Freezer Queen Mini Meal), 7½ oz. 20.8
meat loaf:
    (Banquet), 11 oz. 28.8
    (Freezer Queen Mini Meal), 7 oz. 23.4
    (Morton), 11 oz. 27.7
    (Morton—3-course), 17 oz. 69.4
    (Swanson TV), 10¾ oz. 42.2
    (Swanson TV—3-course), 16½ oz. 52.8
Mexican:
    (Banquet), 16¼ oz. 73.9
    (Patio), 15 oz. 83.3
    (Swanson TV International), 16 oz. 67.3
    (Swanson TV—3-course), 18 oz. 71.3
Mexican combination (Patio), 12 oz. 63.8
noodles and chicken (Swanson TV), 11 oz. 46.1
perch, ocean (Banquet), 8.8 oz. 49.0
perch, ocean (Taste O'Sea), 9 oz. 34.4
Polynesian (Swanson TV International), 11¾ oz. 62.4
pork, loin of (Swanson TV), 10 oz. 40.5
Salisbury steak:
    (Banquet), 11 oz. 21.0
    (Freezer Queen Mini Meal), 6½ oz. 20.1
    (Morton), 11 oz. 24.7
    (Morton—3-course), 17 oz. 66.6
    (Swanson TV—3-course), 16 oz. 46.9
    (Swanson Hungry Man), 17 oz. 63.1
scallops (Taste O'Sea), 8 oz. 44.2
shrimp, fried (Morton), 7¾ oz. 37.3
shrimp, fried (Swanson TV), 8 oz. 41.5
shrimp, fried (Taste O'Sea), 7 oz. 44.7
shrimp patty (Taste O'Sea), 8 oz. 54.7
sole, fillet of (Taste O'Sea), 9 oz. 35.0
spaghetti and meatballs (Banquet), 11½ oz. 57.2
spaghetti and meatballs (Morton), 11 oz. 55.9
spaghetti and meatballs (Swanson TV), 12 oz. 43.5

Frozen Dinners, continued

Swiss steak (Swanson TV), 10 oz. 35.0
tuna (Star Kist), 7 oz. 18.3
turkey:
   (Banquet), 11½ oz. 28.2
   (Morton), 12 oz. 38.6
   (Morton—3-course), 17 oz. 79.4
   (Swanson TV), 11½ oz. 43.7
   (Swanson TV—3-course), 16 oz. 54.5
turkey cutlet (Freezer Queen Mini Meal), 7½ oz. 23.2
veal Parmigiana (Freezer Queen Mini Meal), 8½ oz. 27.0
veal Parmigiana (Swanson TV), 12¼ oz. 47.7

* Note variations in size

FROZEN POT PIES, one whole pie*

See also "Meat & Poultry Entrees, Frozen," "Frozen Dinners,"
"Meat & Poultry Entrees, Canned," etc.

                                                  GRAMS
beef:
   (Banquet), 8 oz. 40.5
   (Banquet—family size), 36 oz. 128.8
   (Morton), 8 oz. 35.1
   (Stouffer's), 10 oz. 36.0
   (Swanson), 8 oz. 38.6
   (Swanson Deep Dish), 16 oz. 56.8
chicken:
   (Banquet), 8 oz. 37.7
   (Morton), 8 oz. 35.4
   (Stouffer's), 10 oz. 39.7
   (Swanson), 8 oz. 40.0
   (Swanson Deep Dish), 16 oz. 55.5
tuna (Banquet), 8 oz. 40.3

Frozen Pot Pies, continued

tuna (Morton), 8 oz. 35.8
tuna (Star Kist), 8 oz. 44.0
turkey:
  (Banquet), 8 oz. 38.0
  (Banquet—family size), 36 oz. 121.1
  (Morton), 8 oz. 34.8
  (Swanson), 8 oz. 37.5
  (Swanson Deep Dish), 16 oz. 63.8

* *Note variations in size*

CHAPTER 12

MEAT, POULTRY, FISH AND SEAFOOD

As you probably know already, most varieties of 100-percent pure meat, poultry and fish contain zero carbohydrate grams—and all varieties of 100-percent pure seafood contain only a small amount of carbohydrate. Within this chapter, you'll find simple specific listings of these no- and low-carbohydrate foods; however, when planning low-gram meals, remember that the key words in the preceding sentence are "100-percent pure." For example, 100-percent pure beef, such as a steak, is carbohydrate-free, but a pure beef frankfurter is not. What's the difference? The difference is that a frankfurter is a processed meat and most processed meats contain fillers which, in turn, contain some carbohydrates. Thus, while a frank—or bologna or salami or dozens of other foods—may be made with pure beef, the "finished" food isn't usually 100-percent pure meat.

Obviously, "combination" dishes such as beef stew and chicken à la king aren't 100-percent pure meat or poultry; therefore, to learn their carbohydrate content, you must 1) keep "score" if you prepare these foods at home, and 2) turn to this chapter if you use processed brand-name varieties. As you review the data here, bear in mind that the figures given for brand-name foods pertain to the specific food and processor listed—or, to put it another way, I'm sorry if your favorite brand of salami or fish cakes is missing, but don't assume that another brand has "about" the same carbohydrate content. Processed meat, poultry and fish may be known by the same name, but, as the figures attest, their composition is frequently as different as night and day.

MEATS & POULTRY, 100-PERCENT PURE*

	GRAMS
meat, raw or cooked, all varieties, all cuts, except bacon and organ meats (see below)	0
poultry, raw or cooked, all varieties, all cuts, except organ meats (see below)	0
bacon, cooked, drained, 4 oz. (about 14 average strips)	3.6
bacon, Canadian, cooked, drained, 4 oz.	.3
organ meats, cooked, four ounces:	
brains, all varieties	.9
gizzard, chicken	.8
gizzard, turkey	1.3
heart, beef	.8
heart, calf	2.0
heart, chicken	.1
heart, lamb	1.1
heart, turkey	.3
kidney, beef	.9
liver, beef	6.0
liver, calf	4.5
liver, chicken	3.5
liver, lamb	3.2
liver, turkey	3.5
sweetbreads, all varieties	0
tongue, beef	.4

organ meats, cooked, continued

tongue, calf 1.2

tongue, lamb 6

* *Data from United States Department of Agriculture. See also pages 113-114 for a definition of "100-percent pure"*

MEAT & POULTRY ENTREES, FROZEN, one whole package*

*See also "Meat & Poultry Entrees, Canned,"
"Frozen Dinners," "Frozen Pot Pies," etc.*

GRAMS

beef:

    and barbecue sauce (Banquet Cookin' Bag), 5 oz. 12.8

    and barbecue sauce (Freezer Queen Cook-In-Pouch), 5 oz. 15.2

    chipped, creamed (Banquet Cookin' Bag), 5 oz. 11.8

    chipped, creamed (Freezer Queen Cook-In-Pouch), 5 oz. 9.0

    chipped, creamed (Stouffer's), 11 oz. 16.5

    and gravy (Banquet Cookin' Bag), 5 oz. 4.3

    and gravy (Banquet Buffet Supper), 32 oz. 21.2

    and gravy (Freezer Queen Cook-In-Pouch), 5 oz. 4.2

    in red wine sauce (Seabrook Farms), 6 oz. 4.9

beef chop suey, see "Chinese Entrees & Side Dishes," page 131

beef chow mein, see "Chinese Entrees & Side Dishes," page 132

beef goulash, w/noodles (Seabrook Farms), 7 oz. 18.9

beef patty, char-broiled, w/mushroom gravy
(Freezer Queen Cook-In-Pouch), 5 oz. 5.0

beef stew (Banquet Buffet Supper), 32 oz. 82.3

beef stew (Lambrecht), 16 oz. 31.2

beef stew (Seabrook Farms), 8 oz. 21.9

beef-stuffed cabbage rolls (Holloway House), 14 oz. 149.0

beef-stuffed green peppers (Holloway House), 14 oz. 135.0

chicken:

    à la king (Banquet Cookin' Bag) 5 oz. 9.0

chicken, continued

  à la king (Freezer Queen Cook-In-Pouch), 5 oz. 6.4

  à la king (Lambrecht), 15 oz. 30.6

  cacciatore (Seabrook Farms), 7 oz. 6.0

  w/cream-style gravy (Freezer Queen Cook-In-Pouch), 5 oz. 5.0

  escalloped, w/noodles (Stouffer's), 11½ oz. 29.7

  fried (Banquet Entree), 14 oz. 41.0

  fried (Banquet), 32 oz. 93.6

  fried (Morton Chicken in a Basket), 32 oz. 100.8

  fried (Swanson), 16 oz. 50.6

  fried (Swanson), 32 oz. 110.2

  fried (Swanson—two ½ chickens), 17¼ oz. 35.8

  fried (Swanson—four ¼ chickens), 17¼ oz. 48.2

  fried, w/shoestring potatoes (Swanson Family Pack), 25 oz. 84.9

  fried, w/whipped potatoes (Swanson TV Entree), 7 oz. 27.0

chicken chow mein, see "Chinese Entrees & Side Dishes," page 131

chicken and dumplings (Banquet Buffet Supper), 32 oz. 110.8

chicken and noodles (Banquet Buffet Supper), 32 oz. 63.9

liver, beef, in onion gravy (Freezer Queen Cook-In-Pouch), 5 oz. ...13.4

meatballs and whipped potatoes, w/gravy
 (Swanson TV Entree), 9¼ oz. 28.4

meat loaf:

  (Kraft Flavor-Frozen), 24 oz. 76.9

  w/tomato sauce (Banquet Cookin' Bag), 5 oz. 10.3

  w/tomato sauce (Freezer Queen Cook-In-Pouch), 5 oz. 11.5

  and whipped potatoes, w/tomato sauce
  (Swanson TV Entree), 9 oz. 20.2

Salisbury steak and gravy:

  (Banquet Cookin' Bag), 5 oz. 7.2

  (Banquet Buffet Supper), 32 oz. 46.5

  (Freezer Queen Cook-In-Pouch), 5 oz. 6.6

  (Holloway House), 14 oz. 37.8

  (Stouffer's), 12 oz. 12.2

  w/crinkle cut potatoes (Swanson TV Entree), 6 oz. 30.5

Sloppy Joe (Banquet Cookin' Bag), 5 oz. 11.0

Swiss steak, w/gravy (Holloway House), 14 oz. 11.2

turkey and gravy:
   (Banquet Cookin' Bag), 5 oz. 5.8
   (Banquet Buffet Supper), 32 oz. 22.0
   (Freezer Queen Cook-In-Pouch), 5 oz. 5.5
   w/whipped potatoes and dressing (Swanson TV Entree), 8¾ oz. ..27.5
veal Parmigiana, w/tomato sauce
   (Freezer Queen Cook-In-Pouch), 5 oz. 14.9
veal Parmigiana, w/tomato sauce (Kraft Flavor-Frozen), 13 oz. 30.6
veal, breaded, w/spaghetti (Swanson TV Entree), 8¼ oz. 24.9

* Note variations in size

MEAT & POULTRY ENTREES, CANNED*, except as noted

See also "Meat & Poultry Entrees, Frozen,"
"Frankfurters, Lunch Meats & Sausages," "Frozen Dinners,"
"Frozen Pot Pies," etc.

                                            GRAMS

beef, eight-ounce serving:
   corned brisket, cooked (Festival Main Meal Meat) 2.0
   corned brisket, cooked (Wilson's Certified Tender Made) 2.0
   creamed, chipped (Swanson) 12.1
   roast, cooked (Festival Main Meal Meat) 0
   roast, cooked (Wilson's Certified Tender Made) 0
   roast, w/gravy (Armour Star) 5.4
beef chop suey, see "Chinese Entrees & Side Dishes," page 131
beef chow mein, see "Chinese Entrees & Side Dishes," page 131
beef goulash (Heinz Minute Meal), 8½-oz. can 20.1
beef goulash (Hormel Mini-Meal), 7½-oz. can 16.4
beef goulash, w/noodles,
   see "Miscellaneous 'Dinner' & Entree Mixes," page 143
beef hash, one cup:
   corned (Armour Star) 20.6

beef hash, continued

   corned (Austex) 22.3

   corned (Broadcast) 22.7

   corned (Hormel Mary Kitchen) 18.0

   corned (Libby's) 29.0

   corned (Libby's Home Style) 35.0

   roast (Hormel Mary Kitchen) 22.0

beef stew, one cup:

   (Armour Star) 13.9

   (Austex) 14.1

   (B & M) 15.2

   (Broadcast) 17.9

   (Dinty Moore) 12.3

   (Heinz) 24.2

   (Libby's) 21.0

   (Swanson) 18.9

chicken:

   à la king (College Inn), 1 cup 8.9

   à la king (Richardson & Robbins), 1 cup 14.4

   à la king (Swanson), 1 cup 13.4

   boned (College Inn), 5-oz. can 0

   boned (Swanson), 5-oz. can 0

   and noodles, w/gravy (Heinz Chicken Noodle Dinner), 1 cup 20.6

chicken chow mein, see "Chinese Entrees & Side Dishes," page 131

chicken fricassee (College Inn), 1 cup 14.8

chicken fricassee (Richardson & Robbins), 1 cup 15.2

chicken stew, one cup:

   (B & M) 15.2

   (James River Smithfield) 22.0

   (Swanson) 19.4

   w/dumplings (Heinz) 22.1

ham, cooked, eight ounces:

   (Armour Star) 0

   (Armour Star Golden) 0

   (Armour Star Parti Style) 2

   (Festival) 2.0

   (Festival Main Meal Meat) 2.1

ham, cooked, canned, continued
(Oscar Mayer Jubilee) 1.6
(Wilson's Certified) 2.0
(Wilson's Certified Tender Made) 2.1
ham, sugar-cured, smoked, prewrapped, eight ounces:
(Amber Brand Smithfield) 8
(Festival Boneless) 2.0
(Morrell's Chef Brand Boneless) 2.2
(Oscar Mayer Jubilee, Boneless) 1.6
(Oscar Mayer Jubilee, Bone-In) 8
ham and lima beans (Austex), 1 cup 25.0
lamb stew (B & M), 1 cup 11.2
meatball stew (Chef Boy-Ar-Dee), 1 cup 14.4
meatballs and gravy (Chef Boy-Ar-Dee), 1 cup 11.3
pork, eight ounces:
loin, smoked, cooked (Festival Main Meal Meat) 2.1
roast, cooked (Festival Main Meal Meat) 0
roast, cooked (Wilson's Certified Tender Made) 0
shoulder butt, smoked, prewrapped (Oscar Mayer Sweet Morsel) ..2.4
Sloppy Joe, one cup:
(Libby's Barbecue Sauce and Beef) 19.2
(Libby's Pizza Sauce and Beef with Pepperoni and Cheese) 19.2
turkey, boned (Swanson), 5-oz. can 0
turkey roast (Festival Main Meal Meat), 8 oz. 0
turkey roast (Wilson's Certified Tender Made), 8 oz. 0
turkey roast, w/dressing (Festival Main Meal Meat), 8 oz. 22.6

* Note variations in size and servings

FRANKFURTERS, LUNCH MEATS & SAUSAGES,
one whole package or can*

See also "Meat, Fish & Poultry Spreads"

To get the most from the data that follows, bear in mind that
franks, lunch meats and sausages are often packaged in uni-

form-size slices or links; therefore, you can usually determine the carbohydrate content of a single piece simply by dividing the content of the whole package by the number of slices or links it contains. For example, if there are 5.4 carbohydrate grams in a full package of bologna and the package contains six uniform slices, it's easy to calculate that one slice has .9 grams of carbohydrate (5.4 divided by 6 equals .9). When meats aren't sliced uniformly, or when you purchase chunks, rolls or rings, you must estimate the size of your serving and then do the required math. In such cases, it's rarely the arithmetic that is hard; it's not "cheating" on your estimate of how much you've eaten. Finally, bear in mind that major processors often market a popular meat in various size packages, and— more important—in different size slices or links. For instance, there is a one-pound package of Oscar Mayer Pure Beef Franks that contains ten links, and also a one-pound package that contains eight links. Both packages contain 16 ounces of the same pure beef franks, but those in the eight-link package are bigger and therefore have a higher carbohydrate content. This point has been made before, but it bears repeating: To keep an accurate count of your carbohydrate intake, you must heed the size as well as the grams per ounce of the foods you eat!

	GRAMS
barbecue loaf (Oscar Mayer Bar-B-Q), 8-oz. pkg.	13.8
beef bologna, see "bologna," page 121	
beef breakfast sausage (Vienna Chubs), 1-lb. pkg.	4.0
beef breakfast sausage (Vienna Links), 8-oz. pkg.	2.0
beef, chopped, canned (Armour Star), 12-oz. can	7.8
beef, chopped, canned (Wilson's Certified Bif), 12-oz. can	6.0
beef, chopped, pressed:	
(Danola Sandwich Beef), 4-oz. pkg.	.9
(Eckrich Slender Sliced), 3-oz. pkg.	1.9
smoked (Buddig), 3-oz. pkg.	.8
smoked (Leo's), 3-oz. pkg.	.4
smoked (Leo's Ripple Pack), 5-oz. pkg.	.7
smoked (Oscar Mayer Thin-Sliced), 4-oz. pkg.	1.5

Frankfurters, Lunch Meats & Sausages, continued

beef, corned (Leo's), 3½-oz. pkg. 3
beef, corned (Vienna), 3½-oz. pkg.** 6
beef, corned, chopped, pressed:
  (Buddig), 3-oz. pkg. 7
  (Leo's), 3-oz. pkg. 3
  (Oscar Mayer Thin-Sliced), 4-oz. pkg. 5
beef, corned, jellied loaf (Oscar Mayer), 8-oz. pkg. 7
beef, dried (Armour Star), 5-oz. jar 0
beef, jellied loaf (Oscar Mayer), 8-oz. pkg. 7
beef pastrami (Leo's), 3½-oz. pkg. 5
beef pastrami (Vienna), 3½-oz. pkg.** 1.0
beef pastrami, chopped, pressed, smoked:
  (Buddig), 3-oz. pkg. 8
  (Leo's), 3-oz. pkg. 4
beef, peppered (Vienna Pepper Beef), 3½-oz. pkg.** 4
beef, roasted (Leo's Beef Roast), 3½-oz. pkg. 1
beef salami, see "salami," page 124
beef, spicy, chopped, pressed, smoked (Leo's), 3-oz. pkg. 4
beef tongue (Vienna), 3½-oz. pkg.** 5
bologna:
  pure beef (Eckrich), 6-oz. pkg. 7.4
  pure beef (Oscar Mayer), 8-oz. pkg.** 4.4
  pure beef (Oscar Mayer Lebanon), 8-oz. pkg. 4.6
  pure beef (Vienna), 6-oz. pkg. 5.4
  all meat (Eckrich), 8-oz. pkg. 9.6
  all meat (Eckrich German), 8-oz. pkg. 5.9
  all meat (Eckrich Sandwich), 8-oz. pkg. 9.6
  all meat (Festival), 8-oz. pkg.** 4.1
  all meat (Morrell Pride), 6-oz. pkg. 3.9
  all meat (Oscar Mayer), 8-oz. pkg.** 4.4
  all meat (Wilson's Certified), 8-oz. pkg. 4.1
  all meat, ring style (Oscar Mayer), 1-lb. ring 14.4
  all meat, ring style (Oscar Mayer Wisconsin), 1-lb. ring 14.4
braunschweiger:
  (Festival), 8-oz. pkg. 5.2

braunschweiger, continued

    (Morrell Pride), 8-oz. pkg. 5.7

    (Oscar Mayer), 9-oz. pkg.** 6.7

    (Wilson's Certified), 8-oz. pkg. 5.2

cervelat, see "Thuringer cervelat," page 124

chicken, breast of, loaf (Eckrich), 6-oz. pkg. 0

chicken, chopped, pressed:

    (Eckrich Slender Sliced), 3-oz. pkg. 1.8

    smoked (Buddig), 3-oz. pkg. 1.1

    smoked (Leo's), 3-oz. pkg. 3

cocktail loaf (Oscar Mayer), 8-oz. pkg. 20.4

corned beef, see "beef, corned," page 121

frankfurters:

    all beef (Eckrich), 1-lb. pkg. 14.0

    all beef (Festival), 1-lb. pkg.** 8.2

    all beef (Wilson's Certified), 1-lb. pkg. 8.2

    pure beef (Oscar Mayer), 1-lb. pkg.** 9.0

    pure beef (Oscar Mayer Machiaeh Brand), 1-lb. pkg. 12.8

    pure beef (Vienna), 1-lb. pkg. 11.1

    pure beef (Vienna Beefsteak Wieners), 1-lb. pkg. 14.0

    pure beef (Vienna Cocktail Franks), 8-oz. pkg. 5.5

    all meat (Armour Star), 1-lb. pkg. 9.1

    all meat (Eckrich), 1-lb. pkg. 14.0

    all meat (Festival Skinless), 1-lb. pkg.** 8.2

    all meat (Morrell Pride), 1-lb. pkg. 17.7

    all meat (Oscar Mayer Wieners), 1-lb. pkg.** 10.0

    all meat (Oscar Mayer Imperial Size Wieners), 1-lb. pkg. 8.5

    all meat (Oscar Mayer Little Wieners), 5½-oz. pkg. 3.0

    all meat (Wilson's Certified Skinless), 1-lb. pkg. 8.2

gourmet loaf (Eckrich), 8-oz. pkg. 11.3

ham, boiled or cooked:

    (Danola Danish), 4-oz. pkg. 0

    (Leo's), 4-oz. pkg. 2

    (Leo's Imported), 4-oz. square or rectangular pkg. 2

    (Plumrose), 4-oz. pkg.** 4

    smoked (Oscar Mayer), 5-oz. pkg.** 5

ham, chopped (Oscar Mayer), 8-oz. pkg. 7.5

Frankfurters, Lunch Meats & Sausages, continued

ham, chopped, canned (Armour Star), 12-oz. can 4.4
ham, chopped, pressed, smoked:
  (Buddig), 3-oz. pkg. 7
  (Eckrich Slender Sliced), 3-oz. pkg. 1.0
  (Leo's), 3-oz. pkg. 4
ham, cured, see "Meat & Poultry Entrees, Canned," page 119
ham, minced (Oscar Mayer), 8-oz. pkg. 5.2
ham and cheese loaf (Oscar Mayer), 8-oz. pkg. 3.3
honey loaf (Eckrich), 8-oz. pkg. 13.9
honey loaf (Oscar Mayer), 8-oz. pkg. 7.9
knackwurst (Oscar Mayer Chubbies), 12-oz. pkg. 5.0
knackwurst (Vienna Knockwurst), 12-oz. pkg. 10.9
liver cheese (Oscar Mayer), 8-oz. pkg. 5.5
liver sausage, ring style (Oscar Mayer), 12-oz. ring 4.8
liverwurst, see "braunschweiger," pages 121-122
luncheon loaf, pressed (Eckrich), 8-oz. pkg. 8.9
luncheon meat, all meat loaf (Oscar Mayer), 8-oz. pkg. 4.1
luncheon meat, canned:
  (Broadcast), 12-oz. can 8.2
  (Spam), 12-oz. can 4.8
  (Treet), 12-oz. can 4.1
  (Wilson's Certified Mor), 12-oz. can 6.4
luncheon roll sausage (Oscar Mayer), 8-oz. pkg. 1.3
luxury loaf (Oscar Mayer), 8-oz. pkg. 6.7
minced roll sausage (Oscar Mayer), 8-oz. pkg. 3.4
New England Brand sausage (Oscar Mayer), 8-oz. pkg. 2.6
old-fashioned loaf (Oscar Mayer), 8-oz. pkg. 15.8
olive loaf (Oscar Mayer), 8-oz. pkg. 17.8
pastrami, see "beef pastrami," page 121
peppered loaf (Eckrich), 8-oz. pkg. 8.8
peppered loaf (Oscar Mayer), 8-oz. pkg. 8.1
pickle and pimiento loaf (Morrell Pride), 6-oz. pkg. 22.6
pickle and pimiento loaf (Oscar Mayer), 8-oz. pkg. 20.0
picnic loaf (Oscar Mayer), 8-oz. pkg. 6.7
Polish sausage, all meat (Oscar Mayer), 12-oz. pkg.** 4.4
Polish sausage, pure beef (Vienna), 12-oz. pkg. 10.2

pork loin, chopped, pressed, smoked (Eckrich), 3-oz. pkg. 1.0
pork sausage, fresh, cooked:
  links (Morrell Pride Tasty Skinless), 12-oz. pkg. 6.3
  links (Oscar Mayer Little Friers), 1-lb. pkg.** 4.8
  patties (Oscar Mayer), 12-oz. box 4.8
  roll (Oscar Mayer), 1-lb. roll 3.2
  roll (Oscar Mayer Hot), 1-lb. roll 3.2
salami:
  pure beef (Oscar Mayer Pure Beef Cotto), 8-oz. pkg. 3.7
  pure beef (Vienna), 6-oz. pkg.** 3.9
  cooked (Eckrich), 8-oz. pkg. 5.4
  cooked (Morrell Pride), 6-oz. pkg. 4.4
  cooked (Oscar Mayer All Meat Cotto), 8-oz. pkg.** 3.5
  cooked (Oscar Mayer Hard Salami), 8-oz. pkg. 3.7
  cooked (Oscar Mayer Salami For Beer), 8-oz. pkg. 1.1
scrapple (Oscar Mayer), 1-lb. can 36.8
smokie link sausage:
  (Eckrich Smokees), 12-oz. pkg.** 12.0
  (Eckrich Smokettes), 10-oz. pkg. 7.2
  (Eckrich Smok-Y-Links), 10-oz. pkg. 7.2
  (Festival Smokies), 12-oz. pkg.** 6.1
  (Oscar Mayer Little Smokies), 5-oz. pkg. 8.0
  (Oscar Mayer Smoked Breakfast Sausage), 5-oz. pkg. 2.8
  w/cheese (Oscar Mayer Cheese Smokies), 12-oz. pkg. 4.0
summer sausage, pure beef (Oscar Mayer), 8-oz. pkg. 2.6
Thuringer cervelat (Oscar Mayer), 8-oz. pkg.** 3.5
turkey breast (Leo's Breast of Turkey), 3½-oz. pkg. 1.1
turkey, chopped, pressed, smoked:
  (Buddig), 3-oz. pkg. 1.2
  (Eckrich Slender Sliced), 3-oz. pkg. 1.9
  (Leo's Breast of Turkey), 3-oz. pkg. 3
  (Leo's Dark Turkey), 3-oz. pkg. 3
Vienna sausage, see "Appetizers, Hors d'Oeuvres & Snacks," page 78

  * *Note variations in size*
 ** *Larger and smaller size packages of this meat contain the same
    number of carbohydrate grams per ounce*

FISH & SEAFOOD, 100-PERCENT PURE*

GRAMS

fish, all varieties, raw or cooked 0
fish roe:
   salmon, raw, 1 oz. 4
   shad, cooked, 4 oz. 2.2
   sturgeon (caviar), granular, 1 oz. 9
   sturgeon (caviar), pressed, 1 oz. 1.4
seafood, four ounces meat:
   abalone, raw 3.9
   abalone, canned 2.6
   clams, hard or round, raw 6.7
   clams, soft, raw 1.5
   crab, fresh, steamed 6
   crayfish (spiny lobster), steamed 1.4
   eel, smoked 0
   frog legs, raw 0
   lobster, fresh, steamed 3
   lobster, canned 3
   mussels, Atlantic or Pacific, raw 3.7
   mussels, Pacific, canned 1.7
   oysters, Eastern, raw 3.9
   oysters, Pacific and Western, raw 7.3
   scallops, bay and sea, steamed 0
   shrimp, raw 5.3
   squid, raw 1.7
   turtle, canned 0

* *Data from United States Department of Agriculture. See also
pages 113-114 for a definition of "100-percent pure"*

FISH & SEAFOOD, FROZEN, one package*

*See also "Fish & Seafood, Canned," "Frozen Dinners"
and "Frozen Pot Pies"*

	GRAMS
clams, breaded, fried (Mrs. Paul's), 5 oz.	41.1
clams, breaded, fried, w/potato puffs (Taste O'Sea Platter), 6½ oz.	55.1
clam sticks, breaded, fried (Mrs. Paul's), 8 oz.	59.5
cod fillets, raw (all brands)	0
crab:	
precooked (Ship Ahoy Alaska King), 8 oz.	1.1
precooked (Wakefield Alaska King), 6 oz.	.8
deviled, precooked (Mrs. Paul's), 6 oz.	34.5
deviled, precooked (Mrs. Paul's Miniatures), 7 oz.	44.1
fish fillets, raw, see individual listings	
fish fillets, precooked (see also individual fish listings):	
buttered, precooked (Mrs. Paul's), 10 oz.	3.1
breaded, French-fried (Gorton's Fish Crisps), 8 oz.	22.0
breaded, fried (Mrs. Paul's), 8 oz.	35.5
fish and chips, precooked:	
(Gorton's English Style), 16 oz.	79.0
(Mrs. Paul's American Style), 14 oz.	94.1
(Swanson English Style Entree), 5 oz.	28.4
fish cakes, breaded, precooked (Mrs. Paul's), 8 oz.	41.8
fish cakes, breaded, precooked (Mrs. Paul's Thins), 10 oz.	72.0
fish puffs, in English batter, precooked (Gorton's), 8 oz.	20.0
fish sticks, breaded, precooked (Gorton's), 8 oz.	16.0
fish sticks, breaded, precooked (Mrs. Paul's), 9 oz.	43.6
flounder fillets, raw (all brands)	0
flounder almondine, precooked (Gorton's), 8 oz.	16.0
halibut fillets, raw (all brands)	0
oysters, raw (Ship Ahoy), 10 oz.	14.1
perch fillets, ocean, raw (all brands)	0
perch portions, breaded, precooked (Gorton's), 11 oz.	12.0
salmon, smoked (Vita Lox), 4 oz.	.1

Fish & Seafood, Frozen, continued

salmon, smoked (Vita Nova Scotia), 4 oz. 9
salmon steak, raw (all brands) 0
scallops:
    raw (Ship Ahoy), 10 oz. 9.4
    in lemon butter, precooked (Gorton's), 9 oz. 10.0
    breaded, French-fried (Gorton's Crisps), 7 oz. 21.0
    breaded, fried (Mrs. Paul's), 7 oz. 45.8
seafood, mixed, w/potato puffs, precooked
(Taste O'Sea Platter), 9 oz. 56.1
shrimp:
    peeled, raw (Chicken of the Sea), 12 oz. 5.1
    peeled, raw (Ship Ahoy), 8 oz. 3.4
    breaded, raw (Chicken of the Sea), 8 oz. 45.2
    breaded, raw (Gorton's), 8 oz. 45.0
    breaded, fried (Mrs. Paul's), 6 oz. 32.8
shrimp cakes, breaded, precooked (Mrs. Paul's), 6 oz. 37.0
shrimp scampi, precooked (Gorton's), 7½ oz. 10.0
sole fillets, raw (all brands) 0
sole fillets, in lemon butter, precooked (Gorton's), 9 oz. 10.0
tuna noodle casserole (Stouffer's), 11½ oz. 34.2

* *Note variations in size*

FISH & SEAFOOD, CANNED OR IN JARS

*See also "Fish & Seafood, Frozen," "Frozen Dinners,"
"Frozen Pot Pies," "Meat, Fish & Poultry Spreads," and
"Appetizers, Hors D'oeuvres & Snacks, Canned"*

GRAMS

anchovies, flat, in oil, canned (Reese), 2-oz. tin 1
clams, canned, one cup:
    whole, meat only (Doxsee) 3.7
    whole, half meat/half liquid (Doxsee) 6.2
    chopped, meat only (Doxsee) 3.8
    chopped, half meat/half liquid (Doxsee) 6.4

clams, w/cocktail sauce, in jars (Sau-Sea), 4-oz. jar 19.1
clams, creamed, w/mushrooms, canned (Snow's), 1 cup 15.4
crab, 7½-ounce can*:
  (Bumble Bee Alaska King) 2.3
  (Icy Point Alaska King) 2.3
  (Pacific Pearl Alaska Snow) 2.7
  (Pillar Rock Alaska King) 2.3
crab, w/cocktail sauce, in jars (Sau-Sea), 4-oz. jar 18.4
fish balls (King Oscar Norwegian), 14-oz. can 10.4
gefilte fish, canned or in jars, one piece**
  (Manischewitz; 2-piece/15½-oz. can) 3.7
  (Manischewitz; 4-piece/27-oz. can) 3.9
  (Mother's; 4-piece/12-oz. jar) 2.6
  (Mother's; 5-piece/27-oz. can) 4.8
  (Manischewitz; 4-piece/1-lb. jar) 2.3
  (Mother's; 4-piece/1-lb. jar) 3.5
  (Mother's; 6-piece/15-oz. jar) 2.2
  (Manischewitz Fishballs; 6-piece/1-lb. jar) 1.6
  (Mother's; 6-piece/1-lb. jar) 2.3
  (Manischewitz; 6-piece/24-oz. jar) 2.7
  (Mother's; 6-piece/24-oz. jar) 3.5
  (Mother's; 8-piece/24-oz. jar) 2.6
  (Manischewitz; 8-piece/2-lb. jar) 2.5
  (Mother's; 8-piece/2-lb. jar) 3.5
  (Manischewitz Fishballs; 12-piece/2-lb. jar) 1.6
  (Mother's; 12-piece/2-lb. jar) 2.3
  whitefish-pike (Manischewitz; 2-piece/15½-oz. can) 3.1
  whitefish-pike (Manischewitz; 4-piece/27-oz. can) 3.4
  whitefish-pike (Manischewitz; 6-piece/1-lb. jar) 1.3
  whitefish-pike (Manischewitz; 12-piece/2-lb. jar) 1.5
herring:
  kippered, canned (King Oscar), 8-oz. can 0
  pickled, in jars (Vita Bismarck), 5-oz. jar 6.7
  pickled, in jars (Vita Cocktail), 8-oz. jar 24.3
  pickled, in jars (Vita Lunch), 8-oz. jar 12.6
  pickled, in jars (Vita Matjes), 8-oz. jar 26.0

herring, continued

    pickled, w/cream sauce, in jars (Vita), 8-oz. jar 17.6

    pickled, w/wine sauce, in jars (Vita Party Snacks), 8-oz. jar 16.4

    pickled, w/wine sauce, in jars (Vita Tastee Bits), 8-oz. jar 24.2

oysters, smoked, in oil, canned (Reese), 3¾-oz. can 12.8

salmon, canned, pink, red, chinook, chum, etc. (all brands) 0

sardines, canned:

    in mustard sauce (Underwood Norwegian), 3¾-oz. can 2.2

    in oil (Crown Norwegian), 3¾-oz. can† ....tr.

    in oil (King Oscar Norwegian), 3¾-oz. can† ....tr.

    in oil (Reese Norwegian Bristlings), 3¾-oz. can† 6

    in oil (Reese Portuguese), 3¾-oz. can† 6

    in oil (Underwood Norwegian), 3¾-oz. can† 3

    in tomato sauce (Del Monte), 3⅓-oz. can 1.4

    in tomato sauce (Eatwell), 15-oz. can 7.2

    in tomato sauce (Underwood Norwegian), 3¾-oz. can 4.1

shrimp, 4½-ounce can††

    (Bumble Bee) 1.0

    (Icy Point Tiny Cocktail) 1.0

    (Pacific Pearl Tiny) 1.4

    (Pillar Rock Tiny Cocktail) 1.0

    (Snow Mist Tiny Cocktail) 1.0

shrimp, w/cocktail sauce, in jars (Sau-Sea), 4-oz. jar 18.0

shrimp, w/cocktail sauce, in jars (Sau-Sea), 6-oz. jar 27.0

tuna, canned, all varieties (all brands) 0

  * *Drained of liquid*
  ** *Drained of liquid or jellied broth*
  † *Drained of oil*
  †† *Drained weight*

MEAT, FISH & POULTRY SPREADS,
one tablespoon, except as noted

	GRAMS
anchovy paste (Crosse & Blackwell)	1.0
beef, corned (The Spreadables), ½ oz.*	1.2

beef, corned (Underwood) ....tr.
braunschweiger (Oscar Mayer) 5
chicken (Swanson), ½ oz.* 2
chicken (Underwood) 5
chicken salad (The Spreadables), ½ oz.* 1.4
chili con carne, w/beans (Oscar Mayer) 2.0
chili con carne, wo/beans (Gebhardt Chili Meat) 8
chili con carne, wo/beans (Oscar Mayer) 1.5
ham, deviled:
   (Amber Brand Smithfield) 0
   (Armour Star) 0
   (Hormel) 2
   (Plumrose) ....tr.
   (Underwood) ....tr.
ham and cheese (Oscar Mayer Roll) 2
ham and cheese (The Spreadables), ½ oz.* 1.3
ham salad (Oscar Mayer) 1.2
ham salad (The Spreadables), ½ oz.* 1.4
liver pâté (Sell's) 5
liverwurst (Underwood) 5
lobster paste** 2
luncheon meat (Spam Spread) 5
luncheon meat, deviled (Deviled Treet) 2
potted meat (Armour Star) 0
potted meat (Libby's) 0
sandwich spread (Oscar Mayer) 1.5
shrimp paste** 2
tongue, potted or deviled** ....tr.
tuna salad (The Spreadables), ½ oz.* 1.3
turkey salad (The Spreadables), ½ oz.* 1.3

 * *Somewhat less than one tablespoon*
** *Canned. Data from United States Department of Agriculture*

CHAPTER 13

CHINESE AND MEXICAN ENTREES AND SIDE DISHES

CHINESE ENTREES & SIDE DISHES

See also "Oriental 'Dinner' Mixes" and "Frozen Dinners"

	GRAMS
Chinese vegetables, one cup:	
(China Beauty)	3.4
(Chun King)	3.2
(La Choy)	4.0
chop suey, eight ounces*, except as noted:	
beef, frozen (Banquet Buffet Supper)	10.0
beef, frozen (Banquet Cookin' Bag), 7-oz. pkg.	8.8
chicken, canned (Mow Sang)	8.0
pork, canned (Mow Sang)	8.0
chop suey vegetables, canned (China Beauty), 1 cup	3.8
chop suey vegetables, canned (La Choy), 1 cup	5.0
chow mein**, canned, one cup:	
beef (Chun King)	11.0
beef (Chun King—divider-pack)	9.2
beef (La Choy)	4.0
beef (La Choy—bi-pack)	7.0
chicken (Chun King)	11.2
chicken (Chun King—divider-pack)	12.4
chicken (La Choy)	5.0

chow mein, canned, continued

    chicken (La Choy—bi-pack) 8.0
    meatless (Chun King) 9.4
    meatless (La Choy) 5.0
    mushroom (Chun King—divider-pack) 8.5
    mushroom (La Choy—bi-pack) 8.0
    pork (Chun King—divider-pack) 7.2
    shrimp (Chun King—divider-pack) 9.1
    shrimp (La Choy) 5.0
    shrimp (La Choy—bi-pack) 8.0
chow mein**, frozen, eight ounces*, except as noted:
    beef (Chun King) 11.2
    chicken (Banquet Buffet Supper) 11.0
    chicken (Banquet Cookin' Bag), 7-oz. pkg. 9.6
    chicken (Chun King) 11.7
    chicken (Temple) 14.0
    chicken, w/rice (Swanson Chinese Style Entree), 8½-oz. pkg. ...24.3
    shrimp (Chun King) 14.4
    shrimp (Temple) 15.0
    vegetable (Temple) 12.0
chow mein noodles, canned (Chun King), 1 cup 24.2
chow mein noodles, canned (La Choy), 1 cup 28.0
chow mein vegetables, canned (Chun King), 1 cup 3.5
egg foo young, frozen (Chun King), 12-oz. pkg. 21.8
egg rolls,
    see "Appetizers, Hors d'Oeuvres & Snacks, Frozen," page 76
pork, sweet and sour, frozen (Chun King), 14-oz. pkg. 55.0
rice, fried, see "Rice, Flavored," page 144
shrimp, w/lobster sauce and rice, frozen (Temple), 12-oz. pkg. 33.0

  * *Approximately one scant cup*
** *Without noodles*

ORIENTAL "DINNER" MIXES*
six-ounce serving**, except as noted

*See also "Chinese Entrees & Side Dishes," "Frozen Dinners"
and "Miscellaneous 'Dinner' & Entree Mixes"*

	GRAMS
chicken chow mein (La Choy)	6.9
egg foo young (La Choy), 3-oz. patty	6.2
pepper steak (La Choy)	7.4
sea food (La Choy)	6.6
sukiyaki (La Choy)	7.7
sweet and sour pork (La Choy)	23.5
teriyaki (La Choy)	5.6

* *Prepared according to package directions*
** *Approximately three-quarters of a cup*

MEXICAN ENTREES & SIDE DISHES
See also "Frozen Dinners"

	GRAMS
beans, Mexican style, see "Vegetables, Canned, Frozen & Mixes,' pages 93, 95	
chili con carne, without beans, canned, one cup:	
(Armour Star)	14.6
(Austex)	12.1
(Gebhardt)	12.5
(Gebhardt Chunky Beef)	14.9
(Gebhardt Longhorn)	17.2
(Old El Paso)	17.5
(Stokely-Van Camp)	13.0
(Wilson's Certified)	14.4
chili con carne, with beans, canned, one cup:	
(Armour Star)	33.8

chili con carne, with beans, canned, continued

  (Austex) 28.0
  (Broadcast) 27.1
  (Gebhardt) 28.8
  (Gebhardt Instant) 24.1
  (Gebhardt Longhorn) 34.2
  (Heinz) 28.2
  (Heinz Minute Meal) 28.2
  (Hormel) 23.8
  (James River Smithfield) 23.9
  (Old El Paso) 34.5
  (Old El Paso Chili Verde y Frijoles) 18.0
  (Stokely-Van Camp) 30.6
  (Swanson) 24.1
  (Wilson's Certified) 24.2

chili con carne, with beans, frozen
  (Banquet Cookin' Bag), 8-oz. pkg.* 21.5

enchiladas:
  beef, canned (Old El Paso), 2.4-oz. piece** 9.0
  beef, frozen (Banquet Cookin' Bag), 3-oz. piece 14.5
  beef, frozen (Patio), 2¾-oz. piece 10.5
  beef, w/Mexican rice, frozen
    (Swanson Mexican Style Entree), 9⅝-oz. pkg. 45.9
  cheese, frozen (Patio), 4-oz. piece 18.9

tacos, beef (Patio), 2¼-oz. piece 15.1

tacos, cocktail size,
  see "Appetizers, Hors d'Oeuvres & Snacks, Frozen," page 77

tamales**:
  canned (Austex), 2-oz. piece 10.7
  canned (Gebhardt), 2-oz. piece 10.0
  canned (Old El Paso), 2-oz. piece 7.5
  canned (Wilson's Certified), 2-oz. piece 8.2
  frozen (Banquet Cookin' Bag), 3-oz. piece 8.8
  in jars (Armour Star), 2-oz. piece 10.8

tortillas, canned (Old El Paso), 5"-diameter piece 8.4

  * *Approximately nine-tenths of a cup*
  ** *Drained of juice or sauce*

CHAPTER 14

PIZZA, PASTA, "DINNER" MIXES AND RICE

PIZZA, one whole pie*, except as noted

See also "Appetizers, Hors d'Oeuvres & Snacks, Frozen"

	GRAMS
cheese:	
frozen (Buitoni Instant), 2 oz.	15.3
frozen (Chef Boy-Ar-Dee), 13½ oz.	116.5
frozen (Chef Boy-Ar-Dee Little), 2½ oz.	23.0
frozen (Jeno's), 13 oz.	108.7
frozen (Jeno's Break 'n Bake), 1 slice**	10.9
frozen (Jeno's Serv-A-Slice), 1 slice**	14.0
frozen (Jeno's Serv-A-Slice Assorted), 1 slice**	14.0
frozen (Jeno's 12 pack), 2 oz.	19.2
frozen (Kraft), 14 oz.	98.8
frozen (Lambrecht), 13 oz.	90.3
frozen (Roman), 2½ oz.	23.3
frozen (Roman), 14 oz.	124.8
mix, prepared† (Chef Boy-Ar-Dee), 15⅜ oz.	130.1
mix, prepared† (Chef Boy-Ar-Dee Mix for Two Pizzas), 14⅜ oz.	120.2
cheeseburger, mix, prepared† (Chef Boy-Ar-Dee), 16⅞ oz.	129.7
hamburger, frozen (Jeno's), 13½ oz.	114.6
hamburger, frozen (Jeno's Break 'n Bake), 1 slice**	11.5

Pizza, continued

pepperoni:

    frozen (Chef Boy-Ar-Dee), 14 oz. 108.6

    frozen (Chef Boy-Ar-Dee Little), 2¾ oz. 23.8

    frozen (Jeno's), 13¼ oz. 95.8

    frozen (Jeno's Break 'n Bake), 1 slice** 9.6

    frozen (Jeno's Serv-A-Slice Assorted), 1 slice** 16.2

    frozen (Roman), 3 oz. 26.0

    frozen (Roman), 14 oz. 116.4

    mix, prepared† (Chef Boy-Ar-Dee), 16⅞ oz. 130.1

sausage:

    frozen (Chef Boy-Ar-Dee), 13¼ oz. 108.0

    frozen (Chef Boy-Ar-Dee Little), 2½ oz. 22.2

    frozen (Jeno's), 13½ oz. 107.3

    frozen (Jeno's Break 'n Bake), 1 slice** 10.7

    frozen (Jeno's Serv-A-Slice), 1 slice** 16.2

    frozen (Jeno's Serv-A-Slice Assorted), 1 slice** 16.2

    frozen (Jeno's 12 Pack), 2 oz. 21.5

    frozen (Kraft), 14½ oz. 99.5

    frozen (Lambrecht), 14 oz. 88.9

    frozen (Roman), 3 oz. 24.9

    frozen (Roman), 14 oz. 116.9

    mxi, prepared† (Chef Boy-Ar-Dee), 16⅞ oz. 127.8

---

* *Note variations in size. Bear in mind that to determine the carbohydrate content of one slice of a whole pizza simply cut the pie into uniform-size slices and then divide the grams in the whole pie by the number of slices. For example, Jeno's thirteen-ounce cheese pizza contains 108.7 carbohydrate grams; if the pie is cut into six uniform-size slices, each slice contains 18.1 grams of carbohydrate*

** *As packaged*

† *According to package directions*

PASTA, PLAIN*

The difference in the carbohydrate content of brand-name plain pasta products is negligible. It is how long you cook these foods, not which brand you use, that affects your carbohydrate intake. What it boils down to (forgive the pun) is that the longer pasta is cooked, the fewer carbohydrate grams it has.

	GRAMS
macaroni (all brands), cooked 8-10 minutes, 1 cup	39.1
macaroni (all brands), cooked 14-20 minutes, 1 cup	32.2
noodles (all brands), cooked about 8 minutes, 1 cup	37.3
spaghetti (all brands), cooked 8-10 minutes, 1 cup	39.1
spaghetti (all brands), cooked 14-20 minutes, 1 cup	32.2

* Data from United States Department of Agriculture

MACARONI, CANNED, FROZEN & MIXES
one cup, except as noted

See also "Pasta, Plain" and "Frozen Dinners"

	GRAMS
and beef, with tomato sauce:	
canned (Chef Boy-Ar-Dee Beefaroni)	32.2
canned (Franco-American)	26.8
frozen (Banquet Buffet Supper), 2-lb. pkg.*	96.6
frozen (Kraft), 11½-oz. pkg.**	47.9
and cheese:	
canned (Franco-American)	26.3
frozen (Banquet Cookin' Bag), 8-oz. pkg.†	36.0
frozen (Banquet Entree), 8-oz. pkg.†	35.6
frozen (Banquet Entree), 20-oz. pkg.††	82.0
frozen (Kraft), 12½-oz. pkg.‡	54.2
frozen (Morton), 8-oz. pkg.†	31.5
frozen (Morton), 20-oz. pkg.††	78.8
frozen (Stouffer's), 12-oz. pkg.‡	43.6
mix, prepared‡‡ (Golden Grain Stir-N-Serv)	44.8
mix, prepared‡‡ (Kraft Dinner)	45.0

macaroni and cheese, continued

mix, prepared‡‡ (Kraft Deluxe Dinner) 44.8

mix, prepared‡‡ (Mac-A-Roni & Cheddar) 41.6

in cheese sauce, canned (Heinz) 27.0

in cheese sauce, canned (MacaroniOs) 23.9

w/cheese flavor sauce, mix, prepared‡‡ (Scallop-A-Roni) 25.5

w/cheese flavor sauce and peas, mix, prepared‡‡
(Noodle-Roni Casserole) 29.4

w/chili flavor sauce, mix, prepared‡‡ (Fiesta Mac-A-Roni) 50.0

w/chili flavor sauce, mix, prepared‡‡
(Kraft Mexican Style Dinner) 54.2

creole style, w/mushrooms, canned (Heinz Minute Meal) 28.4

w/Italian style sauce, mix, prepared‡‡
(Kraft Italian Style Dinner) 46.0

w/tomato-chili sauce, mix, prepared‡‡
(Betty Crocker Macaroni Monte Bello) 38.9

* *Approximately three and three-quarters cups*
** *Approximately one and a third cups*
 † *One scant cup*
†† *Somewhat more than two and a third cups*
 ‡ *Approximately one and a half cups*
‡‡ *According to package directions*

NOODLES, CANNED, IN JARS & MIXES, one cup

*See also "Pasta, Plain," "Frozen Dinners"
and "Miscellaneous 'Dinner' & Entree Mixes"*

GRAMS

w/beef and sauce, canned (Heinz Minute Meal) 18.1

w/beef and sour cream, canned (Hormel Mini Meal), 7½-oz. can* ..15.7

and cheese, mix, prepared** (Kraft Noodle & Cheese Dinner) 49.2

w/cheese sauce and herbs, mix, prepared**
(Noodle-Roni Parmesan) 30.0

w/chicken, in jars (College Inn) 15.8

w/chicken and gravy, canned (Heinz Minute Meal) 20.6

Noodles, Canned, in Jars & Mixes, continued

with chicken meat sauce, mix, prepared**:
    (Kraft Noodle with Chicken Dinner) 46.2
    (Twist-A-Roni) 36.0
with chicken broth sauce and almonds, mix, prepared**:
    (Betty Crocker Noodles Almondine) 52.4
    (Noodle-Roni Chick 'n Almonds) 38.2
with sour cream and cheese sauce, mix, prepared**:
    (Betty Crocker Noodles Romanoff) 52.8
    (Kraft Noodles Romanoff) 44.4
    (Noodle-Roni Romanoff) 39.6
w/soy-celery sauce and almonds, mix, prepared**
    (Betty Crocker Noodles Cantong) 33.1
Stroganoff, see "Miscellaneous 'Dinner' & Entree Mixes," page 142
w/tomato sauce and cheese, mix, prepared**
    (Betty Crocker Noodles Italiano) 55.2

  * *Somewhat more than three-quarters of a cup*
 ** *According to package directions*

SPAGHETTI, CANNED, FROZEN & MIXES
one cup, except as noted

See also "Pasta, Plain" and "Frozen Dinners"

	GRAMS
with meat sauce:	
frozen (Banquet Cookin' Bag), 8-oz. pkg.*	33.8
frozen (Banquet Entree), 8-oz. pkg.*	30.1
frozen (Kraft), 12½-oz. pkg.**	48.9
mix, prepared† (Kraft Deluxe Dinner)	55.0
with tomato sauce:	
canned (Buitoni Twists)	32.3
canned (Stokely-Van Camp)	42.8
mix, prepared† (Kraft Mild American Style Dinner)	53.4

with tomato and cheese sauce:
  canned (Franco-American Italian Style) 33.7
  canned (SpaghettiOs) 36.9
with tomato sauce and cheese:
  canned (Chef Boy-Ar-Dee) 36.6
  canned (Franco-American) 37.9
  canned (Heinz) 30.9
  mix, prepared† (Golden Grain Italiano Dinner) 51.4
  mix, prepared† (Kraft Tangy Italian Style Dinner) 46.4
w/franks, in tomato sauce, canned (Heinz Minute Meal) 28.2
w/franks, in tomato sauce, canned (SpaghettiOs) 27.5
with ground beef, in tomato sauce:
  canned (Chef Boy-Ar-Dee) 32.5
  canned (Chef Boy-Ar-Dee Pizzagetti) 30.3
  canned (Franco-American) 27.3
w/meat and tomato sauce, mix, prepared†
  (Chef Boy-Ar-Dee Dinner) 66.4
with meatballs, in tomato sauce:
  canned (Austex) 31.8
  canned (Buitoni) 24.2
  canned (Chef Boy-Ar-Dee) 31.5
  canned (Chef Boy-Ar-Dee Beefogetti) 29.3
  canned (Franco-American) 26.0
  canned (SpaghettiOs) 24.6
  frozen (Banquet Buffet Supper), 2-lb. pkg.†† 104.0
  frozen (Morton), 8-oz. pkg.* 28.9
  mix, prepared† (Chef Boy-Ar-Dee Dinner) 65.8
w/mushrooms and tomato sauce, mix, prepared†
  (Chef Boy-Ar-Dee Dinner) 68.1

  * One scant cup
 ** Approximately one and a half cups
  † According to package directions
 †† Approximately three and three-quarter cups

RAVIOLI

GRAMS

beef, w/sauce, canned (Chef Boy-Ar-Dee), 1 cup 35.0
beef, wo/sauce, frozen (Kraft), 8 oz. 32.0
cheese:
  w/sauce, canned (Buitoni), 1 cup 31.2
  w/sauce, canned (Chef Boy-Ar-Dee), 1 cup 35.8
  w/sauce, canned (La Rosa), 1 cup 26.6
  w/sauce, canned (Prince), 1 cup 30.7
  wo/sauce, frozen (Buitoni), 8 oz. 26.0
  wo/sauce, frozen (Kraft), 8 oz. 30.8
  wo/sauce, frozen (Roman), 8 oz. 34.9
meat:
  w/sauce, canned (Buitoni), 1 cup 28.3
  w/sauce, canned (La Rosa), 1 cup 33.1
  wo/sauce, frozen (Buitoni Raviolettes), 8 oz. 26.0
  wo/sauce, frozen (Roman), 8 oz. 33.2

LASAGNA & MANICOTTI

GRAMS

lasagna:
  canned (Chef Boy-Ar-Dee), 1 cup 34.3
  frozen (Buitoni), 8 oz. 45.9
  frozen (Roman), 8 oz. 42.8
  frozen (Stouffer's), 8 oz. 24.0
  mix, prepared* (Chef Boy-Ar-Dee Dinner), 1 cup 39.8
  mix, prepared* (Hunt's Skillet Lasagne), 8 oz. 28.2
  mix, prepared* (Jeno's Add 'n Heat Dinner), 8 oz. 22.8
manicotti, wo/sauce, frozen (Buitoni), 10-oz. pkg. 38.1
manicotti, wo/sauce, frozen (Roman), 12-oz. pkg. 58.1

* According to package directions

MISCELLANEOUS "DINNER" & ENTREE MIXES*

See also "Oriental 'Dinner' Mixes," "Macaroni . . .,"
"Noodles . . .," "Spaghetti . . ." and "Rice, Flavored"

Note: Except for the Chef Boy-Ar-Dee and Lipton products in the following listings, these so-called "dinner" and entree mixes call for the consumer to add the main ingredient—meat or poultry—and sometimes other ingredients as well; for example, milk or butter. A typical packaged mix in this category is likely to contain a sauce (or a sauce mix) and/or a seasoning mix, a packet of dry noodles or rice and, in some cases, a can of topping, beans, etc. For the sake of convenience, the carbohydrate content of products listed here is based on the *finished* food, prepared according to package directions. In other words, no matter if a mix is complete as purchased or if it is a mix to which other ingredients must be added, the figure beside it shows the gram content of the food after it has been fully prepared. For convenience too, the generic term for each mix describes the finished food as it is commonly known and/or as it appears on the package.

GRAMS

beef:
    barbecue style (Hunt's Skillet Barbecue), 8.8 oz.** 59.9
    Hawaiian style (Hunt's Skillet Hawaiian), 8 oz.** 30.0
    Mexican style (Hunt's Skillet Mexicana), 8 oz.** 31.4
    Oriental style:
        (Hunt's Skillet Oriental), 8 oz.** 29.1
        (Jeno's Add 'n Heat Oriental Rice Dinner), 8 oz.† 23.1
    pizza style (Hunt's Skillet Pizzaria), 8 oz.** 19.4
    Stroganoff style (Betty Crocker Stroganoff Dinner), 1 cup 41.6
    Stroganoff style (Hunt's Skillet Stroganoff), 8 oz.** 23.4
    Stroganoff style (Jeno's Add 'n Heat Stroganoff Dinner), 1 cup . . .28.6
    Stroganoff style (Lipton Beef Stroganoff Main Dish), 1 cup 38.8
    Stroganoff style (Noodle-Roni Stroganoff), 1 cup 32.8
    Swiss style (Jeno's Add 'n Heat Swiss Burger Dinner), 6 oz.† . . .16.2

Miscellaneous "Dinner" & Entree Mixes, continued

chicken:

    and dressing (Hunt's Skillet Chicken 'n Dressing), 12 oz.** 48.6

    Italian style (Hunt's Skillet Italiano), 14 oz.** 45.5

    and sauce (Lipton Chicken Supreme Main Dish), 1 cup 36.3

    Stroganoff style (Lipton Chicken Stroganoff Main Dish), 1 cup ...36.4

    tetrazzini (Jeno's Add 'n Heat Chicken Noodle Dinner), 10 oz.† ...26.7

    Western style (Hunt's Skillet Chicken Western), 14 oz.** 70.3

goulash, w/meatballs (Chef Boy-Ar-Dee Goulash Dinner), 1 cup 40.5

ham, w/cheese sauce (Lipton Ham Cheddarton Main Dish), 1 cup ..34.9

ham, w/potatoes and cheese sauce
    (Jeno's Add 'n Heat Ham Au Gratin Dinner), 7 oz.† 28.8

meatballs, Stroganoff style
    (Chef Boy-Ar-Dee Stroganoff Dinner), 1 cup 42.4

   * *Prepared according to package directions*
 ** *One quarter of the total prepared yield of the package*
   † *One fifth of the total prepared yield of the package*

RICE, PLAIN, one cup*

See also "Rice, Flavored"

                                   GRAMS

brown, natural (Mahatma) 41.8

brown, natural (River Brand) 41.8

white:

    long grain (Carolina) 40.6

    long grain (Mahatma) 40.6

    long grain, parboiled (Uncle Ben's Converted) 38.0

    medium grain (River Brand) 40.6

    medium grain (Water Maid) 40.6

    precooked (Minute Rice) 39.8

    precooked (Uncle Ben's Quick) 44.1

 * *Cooked, according to package directions*

RICE, FLAVORED, one cup, except as noted

See also "Rice, Plain"

	GRAMS
beef flavor:	
mix, prepared* (Uncle Ben's)	42.6
mix, prepared* (Village Inn)	42.0
w/cracked rice, mix, prepared* (Betty Crocker Rice Keriyaki) ...	39.0
w/vermicelli, mix, prepared* (Minute Rice Rib Roast Mix)	48.4
w/vermicelli, mix, prepared* (Rice-A-Roni)	53.4
w/cheese sauce, mix, prepared* (Betty Crocker Rice Milanese)	48.4
w/cheese sauce and vermicelli, mix, prepared* (Rice-A-Roni)	41.0
chicken flavor:	
mix, prepared* (Uncle Ben's)	42.4
mix, prepared* (Village Inn)	42.0
w/crumb topping, mix, prepared* (Betty Crocker Rice Provence)	57.8
w/vermicelli, mix, prepared* (Minute Rice Drumstick Mix)	44.8
w/vermicelli, mix, prepared* (Rice-A-Roni)	51.4
curry, mix, prepared* (Uncle Ben's)	45.8
curry, mix, prepared* (Village Inn)	42.0
fried, Chinese and Chinese-style:	
canned (Chun King)	46.6
canned (La Choy)	55.0
w/almonds and sauce, frozen (Green Giant)	37.1
w/chicken, canned (Chun King)	56.0
w/chicken, canned (La Choy)	51.0
w/chicken, frozen (Chun King)	35.4
w/meat, frozen (Chun King)	31.9
w/pork, canned (Chun King)	52.9
w/shrimp, canned (Chun King)	50.7
w/shrimp, frozen (Temple)	51.0
w/vermicelli, mix, prepared* (Rice-A-Roni)	49.0
ham flavor, w/vermicelli, mix, prepared* (Rice-A-Roni)	38.0
herb, mix, prepared* (Village Inn)	42.0
w/peas and mushrooms, frozen (Birds Eye), ⅔ pkg.**	43.8

Rice, Flavored, continued

w/peas and mushrooms, in sauce, frozen
(Green Giant Rice Medley) 34.4

w/pepper and parsley, in sauce, frozen
(Green Giant Rice Verdi) 37.8

pilaf, w/mushrooms and onion, in sauce, frozen (Green Giant) 42.2

pilaf, mix, prepared* (Uncle Ben's) 46.8

Spanish:

    canned (Old El Paso) 43.6

    canned (Heinz Minute Meal), 8¾-oz. can** 35.6

    canned (La Rosa) 49.2

    canned (Stokely-Van Camp) 35.0

    frozen (Green Giant) 32.3

    mix, prepared* (Minute Rice) 46.0

    mix, prepared* (Uncle Ben's) 48.0

    mix, prepared* (Village Inn) 42.0

    w/vermicelli, mix, prepared* (Rice-A-Roni) 36.2

turkey flavor, w/vermicelli, mix, prepared* (Rice-A-Roni) 52.0

white and wild, in sauce:

    frozen (Green Giant) 37.7

    mix, prepared* (Carolina) 47.6

    mix, prepared* (Uncle Ben's) 42.8

    mix, prepared* (Village Inn) 42.0

wild, w/vermicelli, mix, prepared* (Rice-A-Roni) 41.4

yellow, mix, prepared* (Village Inn) 42.0

* *According to package directions*
** *Approximately one cup*

CHAPTER 15

SALAD DRESSINGS, FATS AND OILS

SALAD DRESSINGS, one tablespoon

	GRAMS
bacon, mix, prepared* (Lawry's)	1.8
blue cheese:	
bottled (Bernstein)	.7
bottled (Kraft Imperial)	.8
bottled (Kraft Refrigerated)	.8
bottled (Kraft Roka Brand)	.8
bottled (Lawry's)	.8
mix, prepared* (Good Seasons)	1.3
mix, prepared* (Good Seasons Thick 'n Creamy)	.9
mix, prepared* (Lawry's)	.5
(Brockles Special)	1.0
Caesar:	
bottled (Kraft Golden)	.7
bottled (Kraft Imperial)	.6
bottled (Lawry's)	.5
bottled (Seven Seas)	.6
w/garlic-cheese, mix, prepared* (Lawry's)	.7
Canadian, bottled (Lawry's)	.6
cheese-garlic, mix, prepared* (Good Seasons)	.8
cole slaw, bottled (Kraft)	3.4

Salad Dressings, continued

French:
  bottled (Bernstein) 1.5
  bottled (Brockles) 1.3
  bottled (Kraft) 1.9
  bottled (Kraft Casino) 3.6
  bottled (Kraft Catalina) 4.0
  bottled (Kraft Miracle French) 3.1
  bottled (Lawry's) 2.0
  bottled (Lawry's San Francisco) 7
  bottled (Seven Seas Creamy) 1.8
  bottled (Seven Seas Creole) 1.7
  bottled (Wish-bone Deluxe) 2.3
  bottled (Wish-bone Garlic) 3.6
  mix, prepared* (Good Seasons Old Fashion) 5
  mix, prepared* (Good Seasons Riviera) 2.4
  mix, prepared* (Good Seasons Thick 'n Creamy) 1.9
  mix, prepared* (Lawry's Old Fashion) 1.1
fruit, bottled (Kraft) 3.3
garlic, mix, prepared* (Good Seasons) 8
green goddess:
  bottled (Bernstein) 9
  bottled (Kraft) 7
  bottled (Kraft Imperial) 4
  bottled (Lawry's) 7
  bottled (Seven Seas) 5
  bottled (Wish-bone) 1.2
  mix, prepared* (Good Seasons Thick 'n Creamy) 8
  mix, prepared* (Lawry's) 8
Hawaiian, bottled (Lawry's) 5.8
herb and garlic, bottled (Kraft) 4
Italian:
  bottled (Bernstein) 1.0
  bottled (Kraft) 7
  bottled (Lawry's) 8
  bottled (Seven Seas) 7
  bottled (Seven Seas Creamy) 7

Italian, continued

bottled (Seven Seas Viva Italian!) 1.0
bottled (Wish-bone) 7
bottled (Wish-bone Italian Rose) 4
mix, prepared* (Good Seasons) 8
mix, prepared* (Good Seasons Mild) 1.3
mix, prepared* (Good Seasons Thick 'n Creamy) 1.0
mix, prepared* (Lawry's) 8
w/blue cheese, bottled (Seven Seas) 7
w/cheese, bottled (Lawry's) 4.6
w/cheese, mix, prepared* (Good Seasons Cheese Italian) 1.3
w/cheese, mix, prepared* (Lawry's) 8
mayonnaise, in jars:
(Bama) 3
(Best Foods) 2
(Hellmann's) 2
(Kraft) 1
(Saffola) 1
(Wesson) 2
mayonnaise-type, in jars:
(Bama) 1.9
(Miracle Whip) 1.7
(Saffola) 1.2
w/pickle relish (Kraft Salad 'n Sandwich Dressing) 3.0
oil and vinegar, bottled (Kraft) 6
oil and vinegar, bottled (Lawry's Red Wine Vinegar and Oil) 4.2
onion, bottled (Kraft Green Onion) 1.0
onion, bottled (Wish-bone California) 1.0
onion, mix, prepared* (Good Seasons) 8
Parmesan, mix, prepared* (Good Seasons) 7
Roquefort cheese, bottled:
(Bernstein) 6
(Kraft Refrigerated) 8
(Kraft Refrigerated Imperial) 9
(Reese) 1.2
Russian, bottled:
(Kraft) 5.1

Russian salad dressing, bottled, continued
(Kraft Creamy) ... 2.2
(Seven Seas Creamy) ... 1.4
(Wish-bone) ... 7.0
sherry, bottled (Lawry's) ... 1.6
sweet and sour, bottled (Kraft) ... 7.6
Thousand Island:
bottled (Bernstein) 2
bottled (Kraft) ... 2.0
bottled (Kraft Imperial) ... 1.7
bottled (Kraft Pourable) ... 2.4
bottled (Kraft Refrigerated) ... 2.2
bottled (Lawry's) ... 2.0
bottled (Wish-bone) ... 2.5
mix, prepared* (Good Seasons Thick 'n Creamy) ... 1.7
tomato-blue cheese, bottled (Kraft Secret Salad) ... 1.7
tomato-spice, bottled (Seven Seas) ... 5.5
vinaigrette, bottled (Bernstein) ... 5.3

* *According to package directions*

FATS & OILS

	GRAMS
butter, salted or unsalted*, 1 tbsp.	tr.
butter, salted or unsalted*, ½ cup or 1 stick	.5
butter, salted or unsalted*, 1 lb. or 4 sticks	1.8
butter flavoring, imitation (Durkee), 1 tbsp.	2.2
lard*, 1 tbsp.	0
lard*, 1 cup	0
margarine*, 1 tbsp.	tr.
margarine*, 1 cup	.5
margarine*, 1 lb.	1.8
oil, salad or cooking, all varieties*, 1 tbsp.	0
oil, salad or cooking, all varieties*, 1 cup	0
shortening*, 1 cup	0

* *Data from United States Department of Agriculture*

CHAPTER 16

SAUCES, GRAVIES, CONDIMENTS AND RELATED PRODUCTS

SAUCES, half cup, except as noted

See also "Gravies," "Condiments & Seasonings" and "Seasoning & Roasting Mixes"

	GRAMS
à la king, mix, prepared* (Durkee)	6.9
barbecue, bottled or canned:	
(Cattlemen's Regular)	18.0
(Cattlemen's Mild)	39.0
(Cris & Pitt's)	13.6
(Kraft)	33.4
(Open Pit)	50.4
buttered (Gebhardt), 4 oz.	12.8
chicken (Compliment)	27.4
chili (Gebhardt), 4 oz.	12.0
garlic flavor (Cris & Pitt's)	13.6
garlic flavor (Kraft)	34.3
Hawaiian (Chun King)	28.0
hickory smoke flavor (Cattlemen's)	34.0
hickory smoke flavor (Cris & Pitt's)	13.6
hickory smoke flavor (Kraft)	33.4
hickory smoke flavor (Open Pit)	52.0

barbecue sauce, continued

hot (Cris & Pitt's) 13.6
hot (Open Pit Hot 'n Spicy) 50.4
pork (Compliment) 23.5
w/mushroom bits (Open Pit) 48.0
w/onion bits (Cris & Pitt's) 13.6
w/onion bits (Heinz) 33.6
w/onion bits (Kraft) 43.8
w/onion bits (Open Pit) 52.0
w/onion bits, hickory smoke flavor (Heinz) 22.4
barbecue, mix, prepared* (Kraft) 36.4
barbecue glaze, bottled (Bernstein) 31.8
Béarnaise, in jars (Butternut Farm) 6.6
Bordelaise, canned (Betty Crocker) 10.4

cheese:

canned (Betty Crocker) 2.2
mix, prepared* (Durkee) 9.5
mix, prepared* (French's) 8.5
mix, prepared* (Kraft Cheddar) 7.8
mix, prepared* (McCormick) 8.0
chicken, canned (Compliment) 8.7
chili hot dog, canned (Gebhardt), 4 oz. 8.0
chop suey, mix, prepared* (Durkee) 6.0
clam, red, canned (Buitoni) 10.5
clam, white, canned (Buitoni) 10.3

enchilada:

canned (Old El Paso Hot) 9.5
canned (Old El Paso Mild) 9.7
canned (Gebhardt), 4 oz. 8.0
mix, prepared w/tomato paste* (Durkee) 12.4
see also "Seasoning & Roasting Mixes," page 161

Hollandaise:

canned (Betty Crocker) 8.0
in jars (Butternut Farm) 6.6
in jars (Lord Mott's) 7.2
mix, prepared* (Durkee) 7.7

Hollandaise sauce, continued

mix, prepared* (French's) 4.7
mix, prepared* (Kraft) 8.0
mix, prepared* (McCormick) 5.5
Italian, canned (Contadina) 11.6
meat loaf, canned (Compliment) 15.5
mushroom, canned (Betty Crocker) 10.0
Newburg, canned (Betty Crocker) 11.8
Newburg, w/sherry, canned (Snow's) 8.7
pizza, canned (Buitoni) 10.6
pizza, canned (Chef Boy-Ar-Dee) 6.2
pizza, canned (Contadina) 11.3
pork chop, canned (Compliment) 9.7
sandwich, wo/meat, canned (Hunt's Manwich) 15.0
sour cream, mix, prepared*:
(Durkee) 9.1
(French's) 12.8
(Kraft) 16.3
(McCormick) 12.7
spaghetti, meatless:
canned (Buitoni) 11.1
canned (Chef Boy-Ar-Dee) 10.1
canned (La Rosa) 8.5
in jars (Chef Boy-Ar-Dee Homestyle) 14.3
in jars (Heinz) 15.3
in jars (Prince) 12.9
mix, prepared* (Durkee) 10.4
mix, prepared* (French's) 10.7
mix, prepared* (Kraft) 9.8
mix, prepared* (McCormick) 8.7
marinara, canned (Buitoni) 11.4
marinara, canned (La Rosa) 5.8
w/mushrooms, canned (Buitoni) 11.9
w/mushrooms, canned (Chef Boy-Ar-Dee) 14.2
w/mushrooms, canned (Franco-American) 13.3
w/mushrooms, in jars (Chef Boy-Ar-Dee Homestyle) 13.4

spaghetti sauce, meatless, continued

    w/mushrooms, in jars (Heinz) 13.8
    w/mushrooms, in jars (Prince) 12.1
    w/mushrooms, mix, prepared w/tomato paste* (Durkee) 14.0
    w/mushrooms, mix, prepared w/tomato paste* (French's) 9.8
    w/mushrooms, mix, prepared w/tomato paste* (Lawry's) 11.8
spaghetti, with ground beef:
    in jars (Chef Boy-Ar-Dee Homestyle) 11.4
    and tomato, mix, prepared* (Chef Boy-Ar-Dee) 11.3
spaghetti, with meat:
    canned (Buitoni) 10.6
    canned (Chef Boy-Ar-Dee) 12.4
    canned (Franco-American) 9.9
    in jars (Heinz) 15.4
    in jars (Prince) 12.2
    and mushrooms, in jars (Heinz) 14.0
spaghetti, w/meatballs, canned (Chef Boy-Ar-Dee) 12.7
spaghetti, w/meatballs, canned (La Rosa) 12.5
Stroganoff, see "Seasoning & Roasting Mixes," page 162
sweet and sour:
    bottled (Kraft Sauce and Dressing) 61.1
    canned (Contadina) 30.8
    in jars (La Choy) 55.0
    mix, prepared* (Durkee) 22.3
    see also "Condiments & Seasonings," page 159
Swiss steak, brown, canned (Compliment) 5.7
Swiss steak, tomato, canned (Compliment) 6.7
sukiyaki, mix, prepared* (Durkee) 12.6
teriyaki, see "Condiments & Seasonings," page 160
tomato, canned:
    (Contadina) 10.1
    (Del Monte) 6.4
    (Hunt's) 9.0
    (Hunt's Special) 10.9
    (Stokely-Van Camp) 8.5
    w/cheese (Hunt's) 9.9

tomato sauce, continued

 w/herbs (Hunt's) 13.0
 w/mushrooms (Del Monte) 8.5
 w/mushrooms (Hunt's) 9.4
 w/onions (Del Monte) 9.3
 w/onions (Hunt's) 11.7
 w/tomato bits (Del Monte) 10.9
 w/tomato bits (Hunt's) 9.3
tomato paste, see "Tomato Paste & Purée," page 107
tomato purée, see "Tomato Paste & Purée," page 107
white, mix, prepared* (Durkee) 11.7
white, mix, prepared* (Kraft) 11.3

* According to package directions

GRAVIES, half cup

*See also "Sauces," "Condiments & Seasonings,"
and "Seasoning & Roasting Mixes"*

	GRAMS
au jus, mix, prepared* (Durkee)	3.0
au jus, mix, prepared* (French's)	2.3
au jus, mix, prepared* (McCormick)	1.7
beef, canned (Franco-American)	7.7
beef, mix, prepared* (Wyler's)	8.0
brown:	
mix, prepared* (Durkee)	5.3
mix, prepared* (French's)	5.2
mix, prepared* (Kraft)	6.0
mix, prepared* (Lawry's)	8.2
mix, prepared* (McCormick)	6.5
mix, prepared* (Pillsbury)	6.1
herb flavor, mix, prepared* (McCormick)	5.0

brown gravy, continued

    w/onion, canned (Franco-American) 4.9

chicken:

    canned (Franco-American) 6.5

    mix, prepared* (Durkee) 7.1

    mix, prepared* (French's) 7.8

    mix, prepared* (Kraft) 9.1

    mix, prepared* (Lawry's) 6.8

    mix, prepared* (McCormick) 7.0

    mix, prepared* (Pillsbury) 7.2

    mix, prepared* (Wyler's) 8.0

chicken giblet, canned (Franco-American) 5.8

home style, mix, prepared* (Pillsbury) 5.5

mushroom:

    canned (Franco-American) 5.9

    mix, prepared* (Durkee) 5.7

    mix, prepared* (French's) 3.0

    mix, prepared* (Lawry's) 7.8

    mix, prepared* (McCormick) 6.5

    mix, prepared* (Wyler's) 3.0

mustard, mix, prepared* (French's) 3.0

onion:

    mix, prepared* (Durkee) 7.4

    mix, prepared* (French's) 6.2

    mix, prepared* (Kraft) 7.8

    mix, prepared* (McCormick) 7.0

    mix, prepared* (Wyler's) 5.0

pork, mix, prepared* (French's) 4.5

turkey, mix, prepared* (French's) 5.0

turkey, mix, prepared* (McCormick) 7.5

* According to package directions

CONDIMENTS & SEASONINGS,
one tablespoon, except as noted

*See also "Sauces," "Gravies,"
and "Seasoning & Roasting Mixes"*

The carbohydrate content of most spices and many seasonings and dried herbs is negligible—indeed, often nonexistent. Plain table salt, for example, is carbohydrate-free, and a whole teaspoon of plain black pepper has little more than a single gram of carbohydrate. If you're not accustomed to cooking with dried herbs (dill, oregano, thyme, rosemary, etc.), now is a good time to experiment. These super flavor-adders contain a mere trace or less of carbohydrate, but they can work miracles on staple low-gram fare such as fish and poultry.

	GRAMS
bacon bits, imitation:	
(Bac*os)	1.1
(Durkee)	1.5
(McCormick)	5.0
w/onion flakes (Lawry's Baconion)	6.7
bitters (Angostura), ¼ tsp.	.5
capers (Crosse & Blackwell)	1.0
catsup:	
(Del Monte)	4.7
(Heinz)	3.8
(Hunt's)	5.1
(Smucker's)	4.0
(Stokely-Van Camp)	4.5
celery flakes, dehydrated (Wyler's)	tr.
celery salt, see "salt, flavored," page 159	
chili powder (Mexene)	2.4
chili sauce (Del Monte)	4.6
chili sauce (Heinz)	3.8
chutney, Major Grey's (Cresca)	9.0
chutney, Major Grey's (Crosse & Blackwell)	13.1

Condiments & Seasonings, continued

chutney sauce (Spice Islands) 8.0
cocktail sauce:
  seafood (Bernstein) 5.5
  seafood (Crosse & Blackwell) 4.9
  seafood (Del Monte) 5.3
  seafood (Reese) 3.8
  seafood (Sau-Sea) 3.4
  shrimp (Crosse & Blackwell) 4.2
curry powder (Crosse & Blackwell) 4.9
(Durkee Famous Sauce) 2.2
garlic flavoring, liquid (Burton's), ¼ tsp. 2.6
garlic powder (Wyler's), ¼ tsp. ....tr.
garlic salt, see "salt, flavored," page 159
garlic spread, prepared* (Lawry's) 1.1
herbs, blended (Lawry's Pinch of Herbs), ¼ tsp. 2
horseradish:
  (Kraft) 4
  (Tastee) 4
  cream style (Kraft) 2
  dehydrated (Heinz) 5.0
horseradish dressing (Reese) 2.2
hot sauce (Frank's Red Hot), ¼ tsp. ....tr.
hot sauce (Gebhardt), ¼ tsp. ....tr.
hot sauce (Tabasco), ¼ tsp. ....tr.
mayonnaise, see "Salad Dressings," page 148
mayonnaise-type dressing, see "Salad Dressings," page 148
meat-fish-poultry sauce:
  (A.1.) 3.9
  (Cresca O.K. Steak Sauce) 4.0
  (Cresca O.K. Spicy Steak Sauce) 2.5
  (Crosse & Blackwell) 4.8
  (Escoffier Sauce Diable) 5.3
  (Escoffier Sauce Robert) 5.8
  (Heinz 57) 2.6
  (Heinz Savory Sauce) 4.5

meat-fish-poultry sauce, continued
  (H. P.) 3.8
  (Spice Islands Meat Sauce) 5.0
mint jelly (Crosse & Blackwell) 12.8
mint jelly, w/leaves (Reese) 14.5
mint sauce (Crosse & Blackwell) 4.0
mustard, prepared:
  brown (French's Brown 'N Spicy) 1.4
  brown (Gulden's Spicy) 1.0
  brown (Heinz) 1.5
  German-style (Kraft Dusseldorf) 8
  hot (Cresca English) 2.5
  hot (Grey Poupon) 3.3
  hot (Gulden's Diablo) 1.0
  hot (Mister Mustard) 1.9
  yellow (French's) 9
  yellow (Gulden's) 1.0
  yellow (Heinz) 1.5
  yellow (Kraft—in jars) 8
  yellow (Kraft—plastic-squeeze bottle) 9
  w/horseradish (Best Foods) 1.2
  w/horseradish (French's) 1.2
  w/horseradish (Kraft) 9
mustard, mix, prepared* (Durkee Hot) 3.6
mustard sauce (Spice Islands) 3.0
onion flakes, dehydrated (Wyler's) 3.0
onion flavoring, liquid (Burton's), ¼ tsp. .2.6
onion powder (Wyler's), ¼ tsp. ....tr.
onion salt, see "salt, flavored," page 159
onions, minced, dehydrated (Wyler's Instant) ...6.0
parsley flakes, dehydrated (Wyler's) ....tr.
pepper, ¼ teaspoon:
  black** 3
  black, lemon flavor (Durkee) 2
  black, seasoned (Lawry's) 5
  red, chili, dry, crushed** 6

Condiments & Seasonings, continued

peppers, sweet, dehydrated (Wyler's) 3.0
salad seasoning (Durkee) 2.1
salad seasoning, w/cheese (Durkee) 1.2
salad seasoning, w/imitation bacon bits (Durkee Salad Mate) 3.0
salt, table, any amount** 0
salt, flavored, ¼ teaspoon:
  butter, imitation (Durkee) ....tr.
  celery (Wyler's) ....tr.
  garlic (Lawry's) 2
  garlic (Wyler's) ....tr.
  garlic, w/dried parsley (Durkee) 1
  onion (Lawry's) 2
  onion (Wyler's) ....tr.
  seasoned (Durkee) ....tr.
  seasoned (Lawry's) ....tr.
sandwich spread:
  (Bama) 4.8
  (Best Foods) 2.4
  (Hellmann's) 2.4
  (Kraft) 3.0
  (Kraft Salad 'n Sandwich Dressing) 3.0
seasoning, liquid (Gravymaster) 6.5
seasoning, liquid (Maggi) 1
seasoning, mix (G. Washington Brown), 1 packet 1.1
seasoning, mix (G. Washington Golden), 1 packet 6
seasoning, powder (Ac'cent), ¼ tsp. 0
(Shedd's Old Style Sauce Dressing) 1.5
soy sauce (Chun King) 3
soy sauce (La Choy) 9
soy sauce, Japanese sauce (Chun King) 3
sweet and sour sauce (Chun King) 12.6
taco sauce (Gebhardt) 5
taco sauce (Old El Paso) 9
tartar sauce, prepared:
  (Best Foods) 3

tartar sauce, prepared, continued
  (Hellmann's) 3
  (Kraft) .... .7 *
  (Reese) 1.9
  (Seven Seas) 6
tartar sauce, mix, prepared* (Lawry's) 7
teriyaki sauce (Chun King) 1.4
teriyaki sauce, mix, prepared* (Durkee) 1.5
vinegar:
  cider (Heinz) 2
  red (Spice Islands) 5
  rose (Spice Islands) 5
  white (Heinz) 1
  white (Spice Islands) 5
Worcestershire sauce:
  (Crosse & Blackwell) 3.6
  (French's) 1.4
  (Heinz) 2.5
  (Lea & Perrins) 2.0

  * According to package directions
  ** Data from United States Department of Agriculture

SEASONING & ROASTING MIXES, one packet*

See also "Sauces," "Gravies" and "Seasoned Coating Mixes"

The best way—indeed, often the only way—to calculate the carbohydrate content of foods prepared with a seasoning or roasting mix is to 1) determine the number of grams in the dry mix and the number of grams in each of the other ingredients used; 2) combine these figures and then divide the total by the size of your own serving. For example, if you eat one quarter of a seasoning–mix meat loaf that contains a total of 20 grams, it's easy to see that your intake of carbohydrates was 5 grams. Because seasoning mix directions often offer a choice of recipes and/or ingredients, it isn't feasible to list the carbohydrate content of the prepared food here; however, as just outlined, you can easily—and accurately—calculate these figures for yourself.

	GRAMS
beef, ground (Durkee), 1⅛ oz.	19.9
beef, ground, w/onions (French's), 1⅛ oz.	17.0
beef, roast (Roast 'n Boast), 1½ oz.	26.0
beef goulash (Lawry's), 1⅔ oz.	24.1
beef stew, see "stew," page 162	
beef Stroganoff, see "Stroganoff," page 162	
chicken (Roast 'n Boast), 1⅜ oz.	19.3
chili con carne:	
(Durkee), 1¾ oz.	27.2
(French's Chili-O), 1¾ oz.	23.8
(Lawry's), 1⅝ oz.	23.6
(McCormick), 1¼ oz.	13.0
chop suey (Durkee), 1½ oz.	18.6
enchilada (Lawry's), 1⅝ oz.	27.3
enchilada (McCormick), 1½ oz.	24.0
hamburger and meat loaf (McCormick), 1½ oz.	29.0
meat loaf (Lawry's), 3½ oz.	65.2
meat marinade (Durkee), 1 oz.	9.9
meat marinade (McCormick), 1⅛ oz.	17.0
onion burger (McCormick), 1 oz.	16.0
pork (Roast 'n Boast), 1¾ oz.	27.3
rice, fried (Durkee), 1 oz.	10.9
rice, Spanish (Durkee), 1⅝ oz.	24.6
rice, Spanish (Lawry's), 1½ oz.	20.7
Sloppy Joe:	
(Durkee), 1½ oz.	31.5
(French's), 1½ oz.	26.0
(Lawry's), 1½ oz.	27.7
(McCormick), 1-5/16 oz.	25.0

Sloppy Joe, continued

   pizza flavor (Durkee), 1 oz. 12.1

stew:

   (Roast 'n Boast), 1½ oz. 22.6

   beef (Durkee), 1¾ oz. 22.1

   beef (French's), 1⅞ oz. 26.0

   beef (Lawry's), 1-3/5 oz. 24.2

   beef (McCormick), 1½ oz. 19.0

Stroganoff (French's), 1¾ oz. 21.0

Stroganoff, beef (Lawry's), 1½ oz. 23.4

Stroganoff, beef (McCormick), 1½ oz. 26.0

Swiss steak (McCormick), 1 oz. 10.0

taco:

   (Durkee), 1⅛ oz. 14.7

   (French's), 1¾ oz. 24.0

   (Lawry's), 1¼ oz. 21.8

   (McCormick), 1¼ oz. 15.0

tuna casserole (McCormick), 1½ oz. 24.0

* *Note variations in size*

CHAPTER 17

PUDDINGS, CUSTARDS AND GELATINS

PUDDINGS & CUSTARDS, half cup, except as noted

	GRAMS
banana cream:	
canned, ready to serve (Del Monte Pudding Cup)	31.7
cooking mix, prepared* (Jell-O)	29.3
cooking mix, prepared* (My-T-Fine)	32.6
cooking mix, prepared* (Royal)	27.6
instant mix, prepared* (Jell-O)	30.5
instant mix, prepared* (Royal)	30.5
Bavarian cream, cooking mix, prepared* (My-T-Fine)	32.5
butter pecan, cooking mix, prepared* (My-T-Fine)	32.5
butterscotch:	
canned, ready to serve (Betty Crocker)	29.2
canned, ready to serve (Del Monte)	32.6
canned, ready to serve (Hunt's Snack Pack)	30.3
dairy-pack, ready to serve (Sealtest), 4-oz. container	20.6
dairy-pack, ready to serve (Swiss Miss)	18.1
frozen, ready to serve (Cool 'n Creamy)	27.7
in jars, ready to serve (Mott's Snack Pack)	26.7
cooking mix, prepared* (Jell-O)	29.3
cooking mix, prepared* (My-T-Fine)	32.5

butterscotch, continued

cooking mix, prepared* (Royal) 31.8
instant mix, prepared* (Jell-O) 30.5
instant mix, prepared* (Royal) 29.0
caramel, canned, ready to serve (Rich & Ready) 35.1
caramel-nut, instant mix, prepared* (Royal) 29.9
cherry-plum, instant mix, prepared* (Junket Danish Dessert) 33.9
cherry-vanilla, in jars, ready to serve (Mott's Snack Pack) 26.7
chocolate:
    canned, ready to serve (Betty Crocker) 29.8
    canned, ready to serve (Del Monte Pudding Cup) 33.6
    canned, ready to serve (Hunt's Snack Pack) 30.3
    canned, ready to serve (Rich & Ready) 32.9
    dairy-pack, ready to serve (Dannon Bokoo) 27.4
    dairy-pack, ready to serve (Sealtest), 4-oz. container 22.8
    dairy-pack, ready to serve (Swiss Miss Dark) 21.0
    dairy-pack, ready to serve (Swiss Miss Light) 19.6
    frozen, ready to serve (Cool 'n Creamy Dark) 27.7
    frozen, ready to serve (Cool 'n Creamy Light) 27.7
    in jars, ready to serve (Mott's Snack Pack) 26.7
    cooking mix, prepared* (Jell-O) 29.5
    cooking mix, prepared* (My-T-Fine) 31.3
    cooking mix, prepared* (Royal) 30.7
    cooking mix, prepared* (Royal Dark 'N Sweet) 30.5
    instant mix, prepared* (Jell-O) 33.4
    instant mix, prepared* (Jell-O Soft Swirl) 27.0
    instant mix, prepared* (Royal) 31.9
    instant mix, prepared* (Royal Dark 'N Sweet) 31.9
    instant mix, prepared* (Whip 'n Chill) 22.0
chocolate almond, cooking mix, prepared* (My-T-Fine) 31.2
chocolate fudge:
    canned, ready to serve (Betty Crocker) 30.0
    canned, ready to serve (Del Monte Pudding Cup) 32.4
    canned, ready to serve (Hunt's Snack Pack) 28.7
    canned, ready to serve (Rich & Ready) 34.3
    in jars, ready to serve (Mott's Snack Pack) 26.7
    cooking mix, prepared* (Jell-O) 29.5

chocolate fudge, continued

    cooking mix, prepared* (My-T-Fine) 31.2

    instant mix, prepared* (Jell-O) 33.4

chocolate malt, canned, ready to serve (Hunt's Snack Pack) 27.3

chocolate mint, canned, ready to serve (Hunt's Snack Pack) 27.3

coconut, toasted, instant mix, prepared* (Royal) 28.4

coconut cream, cooking mix, prepared* (Jell-O) 25.8

coconut cream, instant mix, prepared* (Jell-O) 29.0

custard:

    Bavarian, cooking mix, prepared* (Rice-A-Roni) 21.7

    egg, dairy-pack, ready to serve (Sealtest), 4-oz. container 24.3

    egg, cooking mix, prepared** (Jell-O) 22.9

    rennet, all flavors except chocolate, mix, prepared* (Junket) ...15.5

    rennet, chocolate, mix, prepared* (Junket) 17.7

custard flavor, cooking mix, prepared* (Royal) 22.5

flan, cooking mix, prepared* (Royal) 20.9

Indian pudding, canned, ready to serve (B & M) 23.6

Junket, see "custard, rennet," above

lemon:

    canned, ready to serve (Betty Crocker) 40.1

    canned, ready to serve (Hunt's Snack Pack) 35.3

    in jars, ready to serve (Mott's Snack Pack) 26.7

    cooking mix, prepared* (Jell-O) 38.8

    cooking mix, prepared* (My-T-Fine) 31.7

    instant mix, prepared* (Jell-O) 30.5

    instant mix, prepared* (Royal) 31.9

    instant mix, prepared* (Whip 'n Chill) 19.3

mocha-nut, instant mix, prepared* (Royal) 31.0

peach, instant mix, prepared* (Jell-O Soft Swirl) 25.8

pineapple cream, instant mix, prepared* (Jell-O) 30.5

pistachio nut, instant mix, prepared* (Royal) 31.2

plum pudding, canned, ready to serve (Crosse & Blackwell), 4 oz. ..62.4

plum pudding, canned, ready to serve (Richardson & Robbins) 68.0

pudding and apricot, canned, ready to serve
(Del Monte Dessert Cup) 34.9

pudding and peach, canned, ready to serve
(Del Monte Dessert Cup) 35.5

pudding and pineapple, canned, ready to serve
(Del Monte Dessert Cup) 34.6

rice, canned, ready to serve (Betty Crocker) 28.0

rice, canned, ready to serve (Hunt's Snack Pack) 27.9

rice, in jars, ready to serve (Lord Mott's) 23.5

strawberry, instant mix, prepared* (Jell-O Soft Swirl) 25.8

strawberry, instant mix, prepared* (Whip 'n Chill) 19.3

tapioca:

  plain, canned, ready to serve (Hunt's Snack Pack) 20.5

  plain, dairy-pack, ready to serve (Sealtest) 21.7

  plain, mix, prepared† (Minute) 20.1

  chocolate, mix, prepared* (Jell-O) 27.6

  chocolate, mix, prepared* (Royal) 29.0

  lemon, mix, prepared* (Jell-O) 27.6

  orange, mix, prepared* (Jell-O) 27.6

  vanilla, mix, prepared* (Jell-O) 27.6

  vanilla, mix, prepared* (My-T-Fine) 25.8

  vanilla, mix, prepared* (Royal) 29.1

vanilla:

  canned, ready to serve (Betty Crocker) 29.5

  canned, ready to serve (Del Monte Pudding Cup) 32.8

  canned, ready to serve (Hunt's Snack Pack) 30.2

  canned, ready to serve (Rich & Ready) 34.4

  dairy-pack, ready to serve (Dannon Bokoo) 27.4

  dairy-pack, ready to serve (Sealtest), 4-oz. container 20.9

  dairy-pack, ready to serve (Swiss Miss) 19.1

  frozen, ready to serve (Cool 'n Creamy) 27.7

  in jars, ready to serve (Mott's Snack Pack) 26.7

  cooking mix, prepared* (Jell-O) 29.3

  cooking mix, prepared* (Jell-O French) 29.3

  cooking mix, prepared* (My-T-Fine) 32.7

  cooking mix, prepared* (Royal) 27.5

  instant mix, prepared* (Jell-O) 30.5

  instant mix, prepared* (Jell-O French) 30.5

  instant mix, prepared* (Jell-O Soft Swirl) 25.8

vanilla pudding, continued

   instant mix, prepared* (Royal) 30.3

   instant mix, prepared* (Whip 'n Chill) 19.3

  * According to package directions—with whole fresh milk when-
     ever directions call for the use of milk
** According to package directions, without egg yolk
  †*According to package directions for "fluffy pudding"*

GELATINS, half cup, except as noted

	GRAMS
unflavored, mix (Knox), 1 envelope	0
all regular flavors, mix, prepared* (Jell-O)	18.2
all wild flavors, mix, prepared* (Jell-O)	17.8
all flavors, mix, prepared* (Jell-O 1-2-3)	18.9
all flavors, mix, prepared* (Jells Best)	18.7
all flavors, mix, prepared* (Royal)	18.4
lemon-lime, w/pineapple, canned, ready to serve (Del Monte Gel Cup)	28.5
orange, w/diced peach, canned, ready to serve (Del Monte Gel Cup)	26.5
strawberry, w/diced peach, canned, ready to serve (Del Monte Gel Cup)	27.4

* According to package directions

CHAPTER 18

CAKES, COOKIES AND SIMILAR BAKED GOODS

DESSERT CAKES, FROZEN, one-sixth of whole cake*

See also "Dessert Cake Mixes," "Coffee Cakes & Other Sweet Baked Goods," and "Specialty Snack Cakes"

	GRAMS
angel food (Howard Johnson's, 9-oz. cake)	26.9
banana (Sara Lee, 14-oz. cake)	35.0
chocolate (Sara Lee, 13½-oz. cake)	36.0
chocolate, German (Morton, 13-oz. cake)	27.6
chocolate, German (Sara Lee, 12½-oz. cake)	27.0
chocolate fudge (Pepperidge Farm, 17-oz. cake)	43.4
coconut (Pepperidge Farm, 17-oz. cake)	46.0
devil's food (Pepperidge Farm, 17-oz. cake)	47.0
devil's food (Sara Lee, 14-oz. cake)	38.3
golden (Pepperidge Farm, 17-oz. cake)	43.6
golden (Sara Lee, 14-oz. cake)	35.0
orange (Sara Lee, 14-oz. cake)	35.0
pound:	
plain (Howard Johnson's, 16-oz. cake)	44.7
plain (Morton, 12-oz. cake)	29.5
plain (Sara Lee, 11¼-oz. cake)	24.4

pound cake, frozen, continued

   chocolate swirl (Sara Lee, 12-oz. cake) 26.3
vanilla (Pepperidge Farm, 17-oz. cake) 47.3

* *Note variations in size*

DESSERT CAKE MIXES*, one-twelfth of whole cake

See also "Cake Frostings," "Dessert Cakes, Frozen," "Coffee Cakes & Other Sweet Baked Goods," etc.

	GRAMS
angel food (Duncan Hines)	30.0
angel food (Swans Down)	29.7
apple cinnamon (Duncan Hines)	35.0
applesauce raisin (Duncan Hines)	28.0
banana (Betty Crocker)	36.6
banana (Duncan Hines Supreme)	35.0
banana (Swans Down)	36.1
caramel (Duncan Hines Supreme)	35.0
cherry (Duncan Hines Supreme)	35.0
cherry chip (Betty Crocker)	37.6
chocolate, deep (Duncan Hines)	34.0
chocolate, German (Betty Crocker)	35.9
chocolate, German (Swans Down)	35.8
chocolate, milk (Betty Crocker)	35.0
chocolate, sour cream (Betty Crocker)	35.4
chocolate, Swiss (Duncan Hines)	34.0
chocolate chip (Swans Down)	37.6
coconut (Duncan Hines Supreme)	35.0
devil's food (Betty Crocker)	35.8
devil's food (Duncan Hines)	35.0
devil's food (Swans Down)	35.3
fudge (Duncan Hines—butter recipe)	35.0
golden (Duncan Hines—butter recipe)	37.0

Dessert Cake Mixes, continued

lemon (Betty Crocker Sunkist) 36.1
lemon (Duncan Hines Supreme) 35.0
lemon flake (Swans Down) 35.8
marble, fudge (Duncan Hines) 35.0
orange (Betty Crocker Sunkist) 36.8
orange (Duncan Hines Supreme) 35.0
pineapple (Duncan Hines Supreme) 35.0
pound (Dromedary) 30.5
spice (Duncan Hines) 35.0
white (Betty Crocker) 35.5
white (Duncan Hines) 36.0
white (Swans Down) 36.2
yellow (Betty Crocker) 35.5
yellow (Duncan Hines) 35.0
yellow (Swans Down) 36.1

* *Prepared, according to package directions, without frosting*

COFFEE CAKES & OTHER SWEET BAKED GOODS

See also "Dessert Cakes, Frozen," "Dessert Cake Mixes," and "Specialty Snack Cakes"

	GRAMS
brownies, packaged (Drake's Brownie Jr.), ⅔-oz. brownie	10.0
brownies, packaged (Hostess), ⅞-oz. brownie	15.5
brownies, mix, prepared*:	
(Duncan Hines Cake Like Brownies), 1 brownie**	21.0
(Duncan Hines Chewy Fudge Brownies), 1 brownie**	20.0
coffee cakes, one-sixth of whole cake†:	
almond, frozen (Sara Lee Coffee Ring, 10-oz. cake)	24.2
apple, frozen (Morton Danish Coffee Cake, 13½-oz. cake)	27.8
apple, frozen (Sara Lee Twist, 13-oz. cake)	23.8
blueberry, frozen (Sara Lee Coffee Ring, 10-oz. cake)	25.0

Coffee Cakes, continued

butter streusel (Sara Lee Coffee Cake, 12½-oz. cake) 30.7

cinnamon, frozen (Morton Melt-A-Way Coffee Cake, 13-oz. cake) . .30.8

cinnamon, mix, prepared* (Aunt Jemima Easy Mix, 14.4-oz. cake). .40.0

cinnamon-nut, frozen (Sara Lee Twist, 12½-oz. cake) 31.4

maple crunch, frozen (Sara Lee Coffee Ring, 10-oz. cake) 27.4

pecan, frozen (Morton Danish Twist, 12-oz. cake) 24.9

pecan, frozen (Sara Lee Coffee Cake, 12½-oz. cake) 27.8

pecan, packaged (Drake's Coffee Ring, 11-oz. cake) 35.2

raspberry, frozen (Sara Lee Coffee Ring, 10-oz. cake) 25.0

cupcakes, mix, prepared* (Flako), 1 cake** 16.0

doughnuts, powdered, packaged (Hostess), 1¼-oz. doughnut 18.2

doughnuts, sugar and spice (Morton Mini), 1 doughnut 8.6

gingerbread, mix, prepared* (Dromedary), 2" x 2" piece 18.8

sweet rolls†:

caramel Danish, prepared* (Pillsbury), 1½-oz. roll 21.0

cinnamon, prepared* (Pillsbury), 1.2-oz. roll 21.0

cinnamon Danish, prepared* (Pillsbury), 1⅜-oz. roll 22.4

honey, frozen (Morton Honey Buns), 2¼-oz. roll 24.8

orange Danish, prepared* (Pillsbury), 1⅜-oz. roll 21.6

 * *According to package directions*
** *Sixteen pieces per prepared recipe*
 † *Note variations in size*

SPECIALTY SNACK CAKES, one piece*

*See also "Coffee Cakes & Other Sweet Baked Goods,"
"Dessert Cakes, Frozen" and "Dessert Cake Mixes"*

	GRAMS
coffee cake, w/topping (Drake's), 2¼ oz.	43.1
coffee cake, w/topping (Drake's Coffee Cake Jr.), 1-1/12 oz.	22.0
devil's food cake, coconut iced (Hostess Sno Balls), 1½ oz.	25.8

devil's food cake, creme filled:

(Drake's Devil Dogs—family pack), 1½ oz. 24.5

devil's food cake, creme filled, continued

(Drake's Devil Dog Sr.—individual pack), 2¼ oz. 38.2

(Drake's Lazy Bones), 9/10 oz. 15.2

(Drake's Swiss Roll), 3 oz. 52.9

(Drake's Yankee Doodles—family pack), 1 oz. 18.0

(Drake's Yankee Doodles—individual pack), 1-1/12 oz. 21.0

(Hostess Suzy Q's), 2¼ oz. 36.5

devil's food cake, creme filled, with chocolate frosting:

(Drake's Creme Cups), 1½ oz. 25.6

(Drake's Ring Ding), 2½ oz. 47.3

(Drake's Ring Ding Jr.—family pack), 1⅓ oz. 21.7

(Drake's Ring Ding Jr.—individual pack), 1¼ oz. 20.3

(Drake's Yodels—family pack), 9/10 oz. 16.3

(Drake's Yodels—individual pack), ⅞ oz. 15.9

(Hostess Big Wheels), 1⅜ oz. 21.6

(Hostess Ding Dong, dark—family pack), 1⅓ oz. 21.0

(Hostess Ding Dong, dark—individual pack), 1⅜ oz. 21.6

(Hostess Ding Dong, milk—family pack), 1⅓ oz. 20.9

(Hostess Ding Dong, milk—individual pack), 1⅜ oz. 21.6

(Hostess Ho Ho—family pack), ⅞ oz. 14.7

(Hostess Ho Ho—individual pack), 9/10 oz. 15.1

(Hostess Cupcakes—family pack), 1⅓ oz. 22.5

(Hostess Cupcakes—individual pack), 1¾ oz. 29.6

devil's food cake, peanut butter filled, with chocolate frosting:

(Drake's Funny Bones—family pack), 1¼ oz. 19.5

(Drake's Funny Bones—individual pack), 1⅜ oz. 21.4

golden cake, creme filled:

(Drake's Crazy Bones), 1 oz. 18.6

(Drake's Sunny Doodles—family pack), 1 oz. 18.7

(Drake's Sunny Doodles—individual pack), 1-1/12 oz. 21.8

orange cake, creme filled, with orange frosting:

(Hostess Cupcakes—family pack), 1⅓ oz. 23.7

(Hostess Cupcakes—individual pack), 1½ oz. 26.7

pound cake (Drake's), 1½ oz. 27.8

pound cake (Drake's Pound Cake Jr.), 1-1/10 oz. 20.5

pound cake (Howard Johnson's Toastees), 1 oz. 16.4

Specialty Snack Cakes, continued

yellow sponge cake, creme filled:

    (Hostess Twinkies—family pack), 1⅓ oz. 22.1

    (Hostess Twinkies—individual pack), 1½ oz. 25.0

* *Note variations in size*

COOKIES, one piece

Bear in mind that commercial cookies are available in literally hundreds of sizes and shapes; therefore, it is difficult—indeed, just about impossible—to accurately compare the carbohydrate gram content of different brands and types. (See "How to Use This Book," pages 19-23.)

	GRAMS
almond flavor (Nabisco Crescent)	5.0
almond flavor (Stella D'Oro Almond Toast)	9.6
almond flavor (Stella D'Oro Breakfast Treats)	15.0
animal crackers:	
(Keebler)	1.8
(Nabisco Barnum's Animals)	2.0
(Sunshine)	1.8
iced (Keebler Party Animals)	7.7
anise flavor (Stella D'Oro Anisette Sponge)	10.0
anise flavor (Stella D'Oro Anisette Toast)	7.8
apple flavor (Keebler Dutch Apple)	4.5
applesauce (Sunshine)	4.4
applesauce, iced (Sunshine)	14.1
arrowroot (National)	3.5
arrowroot (Sunshine)	2.9
brown edge (Nabisco Wafers)	4.1
brown sugar, see "sugar cookies," page 179	
butter flavor:	
(Jacob's Petit Beurre)	19.0

butter flavor, continued

(Nabisco) 3.6
(Pepperidge Farm Bordeaux) 5.1
(Pepperidge Farm Brussels) 4.6
(Pepperidge Farm Cardiff) 2.5
(Pepperidge Farm Lisbon) 3.3
(Pepperidge Farm Venice) 6.3
(Sunshine) 3.5
butterscotch-nut, refrigerated, baked* (Pillsbury) 7.6
Chinese, almond (Stella D'Oro) 21.5
Chinese, fortune (Chun King) 4.6
chocolate:
  (Nabisco Famous Wafers) 4.7
  (Nabisco Snaps) 2.7
  (Stella D'Oro Margherite) 10.6
  (Sunshine Wafers) 2.6
chocolate chip:
  (Chips Ahoy!) 7.5
  (Keebler Old Fashioned) 11.0
  (Keebler Rich 'n' Chips) 8.9
  (Keebler Townhouse) 5.5
  (Nab) 3.9
  (Nabisco) 4.5
  (Nabisco Family Favorites) 4.4
  (Nabisco Snaps) 3.4
  (Pepperidge Farm) 6.2
  (Sunshine) 4.8
  (Sunshine Nuggets) 3.3
  refrigerator, baked* (Pillsbury) 8.2
  coconut flavor (Keebler Coconut Chocolate Drops) 8.5
  coconut flavor (Nabisco) 9.0
chocolate, w/coconut and pecans, iced
  (Keebler German Chocolate) 9.4
chocolate covered sandwich (Keebler Penguin) 13.7
chocolate fudge (Pepperidge Farm Chips) 6.7
chocolate laced (Pepperidge Farm Pirouette) 4.5

Cookies, continued

chocolate nut:
(Pepperidge Farm Brownie) 6.3
   sandwich, fudge creme filled (Pepperidge Farm Rochelle) 9.6
   sandwich, vanilla creme filled (Pepperidge Farm Capri) 9.7
cinnamon (Sunshine Wafers) 3.2
cinnamon graham, see "graham crackers, cinnamon," page 177
cinnamon-spice-vanilla flavor sandwich (Nab Crinkles) 5.6
cinnamon sugar (Pepperidge Farm Old Fashioned) 7.0
cocoa covered (Minarets Cakes) 5.7
coconut:
   (Drake's) 10.6
   (Keebler Bars) 9.2
   (Nabisco Bars) 6.3
   (Nabisco Family Favorites) 2.3
   (Sunshine Bars) 7.6
   caramel, iced (Yum Yums) 10.4
   macaroons, see "macaroons, coconut," page 177
   sandwich, chocolate filled (Pepperidge Farm Tahiti) 8.6
creme sandwiches:
   assorted (Pride) 7.3
   chocolate (Hydrox) 6.7
   chocolate (Keebler Keebies) 7.0
   chocolate (Keebler Opera) 11.6
   chocolate (Oreo) 7.3
   chocolate Oreo; 4-piece/1-oz. pkg.) 5.0
   chocolate (Oreo; 6-piece/1⅝-oz. pkg.) 5.5
   chocolate (Oreo; 6-piece/2⅛-oz. pkg.) 7.1
   chocolate chip (Nabisco) 9.1
   chocolate fudge (Cookie Break) 7.1
   chocolate fudge (Keebler) 13.0
   chocolate fudge (Sunshine) 9.3
   coconut (Orbit) 7.4
   (Keebler Grammys) 6.9
   (Keebler Marigold) 11.6
   lemon (Keebler) 13.8

creme sandwiches, continued

   mint (Mint Hydrox) 6.7
   (Swiss) 6.6
   (Swiss—4-piece/1-oz. pkg.) 4.6
   (Swiss—6-piece/1¾-oz. pkg.) 5.3
   vanilla (Cameo) 10.5
   vanilla (Cookie Break) 7.0
   vanilla (Keebler) 11.9
   vanilla (Keebler French) 13.2
   vanilla (Keebler Opera) 11.6
   vanilla (Social Tea) 7.2
   vanilla (Sunshine Cup Custard) 10.3
   vanilla (Vienna Fingers) 11.1

devil's food:
   (Keebler) 13.9
   (Nab) 13.4
   (Nabisco) 9.8
   (Sunshine Devil's Cake) 10.9

egg biscuits:
   (Stella D'Oro) 6.9
   (Stella D'Oro Jumbo) 7.6
   anise flavor (Stella D'Oro Roman) 19.2
   rum and brandy flavor (Stella D'Oro Roman) 19.2
   sugared (Stella D'Oro) 11.0
   sugared (Stella D'Oro Anginetti) 2.4
   vanilla flavor (Stella D'Oro Roman) 19.2

fig bars:
   (Fig Newtons) 11.2
   (Fig Newtons—variety pack) 20.2
   (Keebler) 14.4
   (Sunshine) 8.8

fruit, iced (Nabisco) 13.5

gingerman (Pepperidge Farm) 5.4

gingersnaps:
   (Keebler) 7.1
   (Nabisco Old Fashioned) 5.4
   (Sunshine—large) 5.7

gingersnaps, continued

  (Sunshine—small) 2.5

  (Zu Zu) 3.0

graham crackers:

  (Keebler Honey) 2.9

  (Nabisco) 5.4

  (Nabisco Honey Maid) 5.3

  (Sunshine) 3.0

  (Sunshine Sugar Honey) 5.2

  almond topped (Keebler Jan Hagel) 6.7

  chocolate covered (Keebler Deluxe) 5.6

  chocolate covered (Milco Dandies) 12.3

  chocolate covered (Nabisco) 7.0

  cocoa covered (Nabisco Fancy) 8.9

  cocoa covered (Pantry) 8.5

  cinnamon (Keebler Cinnamon Crisp) 2.7

  cinnamon (Sunshine Cinnamon Toast) 3.0

  peanut butter covered (Keebler) 5.9

iced (Keebler Swedish Kremes) 12.1

lemon flavor:

  (Keebler Old Fashioned) 11.2

  (Nabisco Jumble Rings) 11.0

  (Nabisco Snaps) 3.1

  (Pepperidge Farm Pirouettes) 4.4

  w/nuts (Pepperidge Farm Crunch) 6.4

macaroons:

  (Sunshine) 12.1

  butter (Sunshine) 4.9

  coconut (Bake Shop) 12.1

  coconut (Sunshine) 12.8

  sandwich (Nabisco) 9.5

marshmallow:

  chocolate covered (Mallomars) 8.6

  chocolate covered (Pinwheels) 20.9

  chocolate covered (Sunshine Kings) 19.6

  chocolate covered (Sunshine Puffs) 10.6

  cocoa covered (Nabisco Puffs) 12.8

peanut butter, continued

    sandwich, chocolate filled (Pepperidge Farm Nassau) 9.2

raisin:

    (Nabisco Fruit Biscuit) 12.3

    (Stella D'Oro Golden Bars) 16.0

    (Sunshine Golden Fruit) 16.2

    iced (Keebler Bars) 10.7

sesame (Stella D'Oro Regina) 6.9

shortcake (Dandy) 7.7

shortbread:

    (Keebler Buttercup) 3.6

    (Keebler Stars) 4.5

    (Lorna Doone) 5.1

    (Lorna Doone—variety pack) 4.8

    (Pepperidge Farm) 8.3

    (Scottie) 4.9

    almond (Keebler Spiced Windmill) 9.2

    cocoa covered (Nabisco Striped) 6.7

    iced (Keebler Fudge Stripes) 7.4

    pecan (Keebler Sandies) 9.2

    pecan (Nabisco) 9.0

(Social Tea Biscuits) 3.6

spice (Nabisco Wafers) 7.4

(Stella D'Oro Angelica Goodies) 14.6

(Stella D'Oro Como Delight) 18.3

sugar:

    (Keebler Giants) 10.8

    (Keebler Old Fashioned) 12.4

    (Nabisco Rings) 10.7

    (Pepperidge Farm) 7.0

    refrigerator, baked* (Pillsbury) 7.7

    brown (Nabisco Family Favorites) 3.0

    brown (Pepperidge Farm) 6.9

sugar wafers:

    (Biscos) 2.5

    (Biscos—variety pack) 5.8

    (Bisco Waffle Cremes) 6.0

sugar wafers, continued

(Kremelined) 6.2
(Sunshine) 6.8
(Sunshine Clover Leaves) 6.2
chocolate (Keebler Krisp Kreem) 3.5
chocolate covered (Milco) 10.1
chocolate covered (Sunshine Ice Box) 4.8
cocoa covered (Nabisco Creme Wafer Sticks) 5.9
strawberry (Keebler Krisp Kreem) 3.7
vanilla (Keebler Krisp Kreem) 3.7
vanilla:
(Keebler Wafers) 2.5
(Nabisco Snaps) 2.3
(Nilla Wafers) 2.9
(Pepperidge Farm Pirouettes) 4.4
(Stella D'Oro Margherite) 10.5
(Sunshine Wafers) 2.1
sandwich, chocolate filled (Pepperidge Farm Lido) 10.0
sandwich, chocolate filled (Pepperidge Farm Milano) 7.2
sandwich, chocolate-mint filled
    (Pepperidge Farm Mint Milano) 8.4
wafer, chocolate coated (Pepperidge Farm Orleans) 3.5

* According to package directions

CHAPTER 19

PIES AND PASTRIES

FROZEN DESSERT PIES,
one-sixth of whole pie, except as noted

See also "Specialty Snack Pies" and "Specialty Pastries"

	GRAMS
cream varieties, eight-inch diameter*:	
banana (Banquet, 14-oz. pie)	23.3
banana (Morton, 14-oz. pie)	23.3
banana (Mrs. Smith's, 13-oz. pie)	23.2
butterscotch (Banquet, 14-oz. pie)	25.2
chocolate (Banquet, 14-oz. pie)	26.6
chocolate (Mrs. Smith's, 13-oz. pie)	25.5
chocolate-nut (Kraft, 16¾-oz. pie)	30.5
coconut (Banquet, 14-oz. pie)	22.6
coconut (Morton, 14-oz. pie)	24.3
coconut (Mrs. Smith's, 13-oz. pie)	24.5
key lime (Banquet, 14-oz. pie)	25.7
lemon (Banquet, 14-oz. pie)	23.8
lemon (Morton, 14-oz. pie)	24.3
lemon (Mrs. Smith's, 13-oz. pie)	22.7
mint (Kraft Mint Mist, 13-oz. pie)	24.6
Neapolitan (Banquet, 14-oz. pie)	25.4
Neapolitan (Morton, 14-oz. pie)	23.6

* Remember: the data pertains to one-sixth of the whole pie

cream varieties, eight-inch diameter, continued

Neapolitan (Mrs. Smith's, 13-oz. pie) 25.5
peppermint, pink (Kraft, 13-oz. pie) 26.9
strawberry (Banquet, 14-oz. pie) 23.8
strawberry (Morton, 14-oz. pie) 21.6
strawberry (Mrs. Smith's, 13-oz. pie) 23.7
fruit and custard varieties, eight-inch diameter*:
apple (Banquet, 20-oz. pie) 33.0
apple (Morton, 20-oz. pie) 33.6
apple (Morton, 24-oz. pie) 40.1
apple (Mrs. Smith's, 26-oz. pie) 42.0
apple, Dutch, crumb (Mrs. Smith's, 26-oz. pie) 47.2
apple, Dutch tart (Mrs. Smith's, 26-oz. pie) 43.8
blackberry (Banquet, 20-oz. pie) 37.0
blackberry (Mrs. Smith's, 26-oz. pie) 39.2
blueberry (Banquet, 20-oz. pie) 37.2
blueberry (Morton, 20-oz. pie) 33.5
blueberry (Mrs. Smith's, 26-oz. pie) 39.2
boysenberry (Banquet, 20-oz. pie) 36.2
cherry (Banquet, 20-oz. pie) 33.5
cherry (Morton, 20-oz. pie) 35.7
cherry (Morton, 24-oz. pie) 39.6
cherry (Mrs. Smith's, 26-oz. pie) 35.3
custard (Banquet, 20-oz. pie) 27.5
custard (Mrs. Smith's, 25-oz. pie) 28.8
custard, coconut (Banquet, 20-oz. pie) 26.5
custard, coconut (Morton, 20-oz. pie) 27.7
custard, coconut (Mrs. Smith's, 25-oz. pie) 31.7
lemon (Mrs. Smith's, 26-oz. pie) 46.3
lemon meringue (Mrs. Smith's, 20-oz. pie) 41.0
mince (Banquet, 20-oz. pie) 41.8
mince (Morton, 20-oz. pie) 35.8
mince (Mrs. Smith's, 26-oz. pie) 48.2
peach (Banquet, 20-oz. pie) 30.3
peach (Morton, 20-oz. pie) 34.9
peach (Morton, 24-oz. pie) 44.3
peach (Mrs. Smith's, 26-oz. pie) 42.0

* *Remember: the data pertains to one-sixth of the whole pie*

fruit and custard varieties, eight-inch diameter, continued

pecan (Morton, 20-oz. pie) 49.4
pecan (Mrs. Smith's, 24-oz. pie) 52.0
pineapple (Mrs. Smith's, 26-oz. pie) 43.8
pineapple cheese (Mrs. Smith's, 26-oz. pie) 36.3
pumpkin (Banquet, 20-oz. pie) 31.0
pumpkin (Morton, 20-oz. pie) 26.2
pumpkin custard (Mrs. Smith's, 26-oz. pie) 33.5
raisin (Mrs. Smith's, 26-oz. pie) 42.0
strawberry (Morton, 20-oz. pie) 36.8
strawberry-rhubarb (Mrs. Smith's, 26-oz. pie) 45.8

fruit varieties, nine-inch diameter*:

apple (Mrs. Smith's Old Fashioned, 38-oz. pie) 74.7
blackberry (Mrs. Smith's Old Fashioned, 38-oz. pie) 65.2
blueberry (Mrs. Smith's Old Fashioned, 38-oz. pie) 65.2
cherry (Mrs. Smith's Old Fashioned, 38-oz. pie) 66.2
peach (Mrs. Smith's Old Fashioned, 38-oz. pie) 73.7
strawberry-rhubarb (Mrs. Smith's Old Fashioned, 38-oz. pie) 58.7

fruit and custard varieties,
ten-inch diameter, one-eighth of whole pie**:

apple (Banquet, 46-oz. pie) 56.9
apple (Morton Home Style, 46-oz. pie) 57.4
apple (Mrs. Smith's Golden Deluxe, 46-oz. pie) 55.3
apple crumb (Mrs. Smith's Golden Deluxe, 46-oz. pie) 62.4
blackberry (Banquet, 46-oz. pie) 63.8
blackberry (Mrs. Smith's Golden Deluxe, 46-oz. pie) 51.4
blueberry (Banquet, 46-oz. pie) 64.1
blueberry (Morton Home Style, 46-oz. pie) 56.5
blueberry (Mrs. Smith's Golden Deluxe, 46-oz. pie) 51.4
cherry (Banquet, 46-oz. pie) 57.8
cherry (Morton Home Style, 46-oz. pie) 63.1
cherry (Mrs. Smith's Golden Deluxe, 46-oz. pie) 46.4
custard (Banquet, 46-oz. pie) 47.4
custard, coconut (Banquet, 46-oz. pie) 45.7
custard, coconut (Morton Home Style, 46-oz. pie) 60.3
custard, coconut (Mrs. Smith's Golden Deluxe, 44-oz. pie) 39.6

* *Remember: the data pertains to one-sixth of the whole pie*
** *Remember: the data pertains to one-eighth of the whole pie*

fruit and custard pies, ten-inch diameter**, continued

lemon meringue (Mrs. Smith's Golden Deluxe, 36-oz. pie) 54.3
mince (Banquet, 46-oz. pie) 72.2
mince (Morton Home Style, 46-oz. pie) 58.4
mince (Mrs. Smith's Golden Deluxe, 46-oz. pie) 63.4
peach (Banquet, 46-oz. pie) 52.3
peach (Morton Home Style, 46-oz. pie) 60.8
peach (Mrs. Smith's Golden Deluxe, 46-oz. pie) 55.3
pecan (Morton Home Style, 46-oz. pie) 87.5
pecan (Mrs. Smith's Golden Deluxe, 36-oz. pie) 57.4
pumpkin (Banquet, 46-oz. pie) 53.5
pumpkin (Morton Home Style, 46-oz. pie) 61.1
pumpkin custard (Mrs. Smith's Golden Deluxe, 44-oz. pie) 43.3
pineapple (Morton Home Style, 46-oz. pie) 60.5
pineapple cheese (Mrs. Smith's Golden Deluxe, 46-oz. pie) 80.8
strawberry-rhubarb (Morton Home Style, 46-oz. pie) 68.8
strawberry-rhubarb (Mrs. Smith's Golden Deluxe, 46-oz. pie) ...60.6

** Remember: the data pertains to one-eighth of the whole pie

PASTRY SHELLS & PIE CRUSTS

GRAMS

pastry shells, ready-to-use (Stella D'Oro), 8/10-oz. shell 16.2
patty shells, frozen (Pepperidge Farm), 1⅔-oz. shell 18.1
pie crusts, frozen:
    plain, 8" diameter (Morton), 1 pkg.* 116.0
    plain, 8" diameter (Mrs. Smith's), 1 pkg.* 124.0
    honey graham, 8" diameter (Mrs. Smith's), 1 pkg.* 158.0
    plain, 9" diameter (Mrs. Smith's), 1 pkg.* 182.0
    plain, 10" diameter (Mrs. Smith's), 1 pkg.* 204.0
    honey graham, 10" diameter (Mrs. Smith's), 1 pkg.* 226.0
pie crusts, mix, prepared** (Flako), single 9" crust 72.0

* Two shells per package
** According to package directions

SPECIALTY PASTRIES:
PIE-TARTS, TURNOVERS, STRUDELS, ETC.
one whole piece*, except as noted

See also "Frozen Dessert Pies," and " 'Toaster' Pastries"

	GRAMS
dumplings, apple, frozen (Pepperidge Farm), 3.1 oz.	30.7
dumplings, peach, frozen (Pepperidge Farm), 3.1 oz.	34.6
pie-tarts:	
apple, frozen (Pepperidge Farm), 2⅞ oz.	32.8
blueberry, frozen (Pepperidge Farm), 2⅞ oz.	34.5
cherry, frozen (Pepperidge Farm), 2⅞ oz.	34.3
chocolate, frozen (Pepperidge Farm), 2⅞ oz.	35.2
coconut creme, frozen (Pepperidge Farm), 2⅞ oz.	29.0
turnovers:	
apple, frozen (Pepperidge Farm), 3.1 oz.	30.2
apple, refrigerated (Pillsbury), 1¾ oz.	32.0
blueberry, frozen (Pepperidge Farm), 3.1 oz.	32.0
cherry, frozen (Pepperidge Farm), 3.1 oz.	30.3
cherry, refrigerated (Pillsbury), 1¾ oz.	20.5
lemon, frozen (Pepperidge Farm), 3.1 oz.	33.1
peach, frozen (Pepperidge Farm), 3.1 oz.	33.4
raspberry, frozen (Pepperidge Farm), 3.1 oz.	36.9
strawberry, frozen (Pepperidge Farm), 3.1 oz.	34.5
strudels, one-sixth of 14-ounce strudel:	
apple, frozen (Pepperidge Farm)	26.0
blueberry, frozen (Pepperidge Farm)	28.4
cherry, frozen (Pepperidge Farm)	26.8
pineapple-cheese, frozen (Pepperidge Farm)	21.2

* Note variations in size

SPECIALTY SNACK PIES, one complete package*

See also "Frozen Dessert Pies" and "Specialty Pastries"

	GRAMS
apple (Drake Fruit Pie), 4 oz.	55.9
apple (Hostess Fruit Pie), 4½ oz.	60.4
cherry (Drake Fruit Pie), 4 oz.	53.4
cherry (Hostess Fruit Pie), 4½ oz.	56.0
lemon (Hostess Fruit Pie), 4½ oz.	53.9

* *Note variations in size*

"TOASTER" PASTRIES, one tart*

See also "Specialty Pastries"

	GRAMS
all fruit flavors (Toast 'em Danka Danish), 1½ oz.	24.5
all fruit flavors, except frosted (Toast 'em Pop-Ups), 1¾ oz.	32.5
all fruit flavors (Kellogg's Danish Go-Rounds), 2 oz.	41.6
all fruit flavors, except frosted (Kellogg's Pop Tarts), 1.8 oz.	36.9
all fruit frosted flavors (Toast 'em Pop-Ups), 1.8 oz.	37.4
all fruit frosted flavors (Kellogg's Pop Tarts), 1.8 oz.	36.6
apple (Nabisco Toastettes), 1.7 oz.	32.3
blueberry (Nabisco Toastettes), 1.7 oz.	33.0
brown sugar-cinnamon (Kellogg's Pop Tarts), 1.8 oz.	34.6
brown sugar-cinnamon (Nabisco Toastettes), 1.7 oz.	31.3
cherry (Nabisco Toastettes), 1.7 oz.	32.7
chocolate, frosted (Kellogg's Pop Tarts), 1.8 oz.	34.2
orange marmalade (Nabisco Toastettes), 1.7 oz.	32.1
peach (Nabisco Toastettes), 1.7 oz.	32.7
strawberry (Nabisco Toastettes), 1.7 oz.	32.7

* *Note variations in size*

CHAPTER 20

PEANUT BUTTER, JELLIES AND JAMS

PEANUT BUTTER, one tablespoon

	GRAMS
(Bama)	3.6
(Big Top)	3.0
(Jif)	3.0
(Peter Pan)	3.9
(Planters)	2.9
(Skippy, Chunk)	2.3
(Skippy, Creamy)	2.3
(Smucker's)	4.6
and grape jelly (Smucker's Goober)	9.6

JAMS, JELLIES & PRESERVES, one tablespoon

	GRAMS
butters:	
apple (Bama)	7.7
apple (Ma Brown)	10.7
apple (Musselman's)	8.4
apple (Smucker's)	9.8
peach (Smucker's)	11.6

jams:

    all flavors, except apricot, peach, pear and plum (Bama) 13.5

    apricot (Bama) 12.7

    grape (Kraft) 12.9

    grape (Welch's Grapelade) 13.8

    peach (Bama) 12.7

    pear (Bama) 12.7

    plum (Bama) 12.7

    strawberry (Musselman's) 14.1

jellies:

    all flavors (Bama) 12.7

    all flavors (Crosse & Blackwell) 12.8

    all flavors (Kraft) 11.4

    all flavors (Ma Brown) 11.3

    all flavors (Musselman's) 13.5

    all flavors (Smucker's) 12.3

    all flavors (Welch's) 12.5

marmalade:

    all flavors (Crosse & Blackwell) 14.9

    orange (Bama) 13.5

    orange (Kraft) 12.8

    orange (Ma Brown) 11.3

    (Musselman's) 13.0

    (Welch's) 13.8

preserves:

    all flavors, except apricot, peach, pear and plum (Bama) 13.5

    all flavors (Crosse & Blackwell) 14.8

    all flavors (Ma Brown) 11.3

    all flavors (Smucker's) 13.5

    all flavors, except peach (Welch's) 13.8

    apricot (Bama) 12.7

    blackberry (Kraft) 13.1

    blueberry, wild (Reese) 14.1

    grape (Kraft) 12.2

    peach (Bama) 12.7

CHAPTER 21

SYRUPS, TOPPINGS AND RELATED PRODUCTS

HONEY, MOLASSES, SUGAR & SYRUPS, one tablespoon

See also "Dessert Toppings" and "Sweet Flavorings"

	GRAMS
honey, strained or extracted*	17.3
molasses, dark (Brer Rabbit)	13.3
molasses, light (Brer Rabbit)	14.6
sugar, brown (all brands)	13.4
sugar, granulated (all brands)	12.0
sugar, powdered (all brands)	8.0
syrups:	
chocolate flavor (Hershey)	12.4
corn, dark (Karo)	14.6
corn, light (Karo)	14.6
fruit (Smucker's)	10.8
maple, pure (Cary's)	14.3
maple, blended (Log Cabin)	12.2
maple, blended (Vermont Maid)	13.4
maple flavor:	
(Aunt Jemima)	13.0
(Bama)	13.2
(Happy Jack Pancake)	13.2
(Karo Pancake-Waffle)	14.6

maple flavor syrups, continued

    (Log Cabin Country Kitchen) 13.1
    (Smucker's Pancake) 10.8
    w/butter (Log Cabin Buttered) 12.7
    w/honey (Log Cabin Maple Honey) 14.0

* *Data from United States Department of Agriculture*

DESSERT TOPPINGS, one tablespoon
See also "Honey, Molasses, Sugar & Syrups"

	GRAMS
butterscotch (Kraft)	12.3
butterscotch (Smucker's)	15.0
caramel (Kraft)	13.0
caramel (Smucker's)	14.8
caramel, chocolate (Kraft)	11.9
chocolate flavor (Kraft)	11.8
chocolate flavor (Smucker's)	13.4
chocolate fudge (Hershey)	9.7
chocolate fudge (Kraft)	9.8
chocolate fudge (Smucker's)	13.4
cream, whipped, aerosol canned (Reddi-Wip)	.4
cream, whipped, aerosol canned (Sealtest Zip Whipt)	.6
hard sauce (Crosse & Blackwell)	8.3
marshmallow creme (Kraft)	5.2
pecans, in syrup (Kraft)	9.2
pecans, in syrup (Smucker's)	8.0
pineapple (Kraft)	13.8
pineapple (Smucker's)	14.0
spoonmallow (Kraft)	8.6
strawberry (Kraft)	12.7
walnuts, in syrup (Kraft)	9.1
walnuts, in syrup (Smucker's)	8.2

Dessert Toppings, continued
whip, non-dairy:
    aerosol canned (Kraft) 5
    aerosol canned (Lucky Whip) 4
    aerosol canned (Reddi-Wip) 4
    aerosol canned (Sealtest Big Top) 3
    frozen (Cool Whip) 1.1
    frozen (Pet) 1.1
    mix, prepared* (Dream Whip) 1.2
    mix, prepared* (Lucky Whip) 1.2

* *According to package directions*

SWEET FLAVORINGS, one teaspoon

See also "Dessert Toppings"
and "Honey, Molasses, Sugar & Syrups"

	GRAMS
almond, extract, pure (Durkee)	3.3
anise extract, imitation (Durkee)	4.0
banana extract, imitation (Durkee)	3.8
black walnut flavor, imitation (Durkee)	1.0
brandy extract, imitation (Durkee)	3.8
cherry extract, pure (Burton's)	2.2
coconut flavor, imitation (Durkee)	2.0
coffee flavor, pure (Burton's)	2.1
grenadine syrup:	
nonalcoholic (Garnier)	4.3
nonalcoholic (Giroux)	4.2
nonalcoholic (Holland House)	3.8
25 proof (Leroux)	2.5
lemon extract, imitation (Durkee)	4.3
maple extract, imitation (Durkee)	1.5

Sweet Flavorings, continued

mocha extract, imitation (Durkee) 3.5
orange extract, imitation (Durkee) 4.0
orgeat syrup (Julius Wile) 4.3
peppermint extract, pure (Burton's) 3.0
peppermint extract, imitation (Durkee) 3.8
pineapple flavor, pure (Burton's) 3.0
raspberry extract, pure (Burton's) 2.0
raspberry extract, imitation (Burton's) 2.6
rose extract, pure (Burton's) 2.2
rum extract, imitation (Burton's) 2.7
rum extract, imitation (Durkee) 3.5
strawberry extract, pure (Burton's) 2.4
strawberry extract, imitation (Durkee) 3.0
vanilla extract, pure (Burnett's) 2.3
vanilla extract, pure (Durkee) 2.0
vanilla extract, imitation (Durkee) 8
vanilla extract, imitation (Gold Medal) 1

SWEET BAKING INGREDIENTS, one ounce

	GRAMS
butterscotch (Nestlé Morsels)	17.0
chocolate:	
pre-melted (Nestlé Choco-Bake)	13.5
milk (Hershey Chips)	17.2
milk (Nestlé Morsels)	17.3
sweet (Baker's German)	16.9
semisweet (Baker's)	16.2
semisweet (Baker's Chips)	19.0
semisweet (Ghirardelli Chips)	17.8
semisweet (Hershey Chips)	17.2
semisweet (Nestlé Morsels)	18.1
semisweet, mint flavor (Nestlé Morsels)	18.1

baking chocolate, continued

unsweetened (Baker's) 7.7
unsweetened (Hershey Baking) 6.6
coconut, dried:
(Baker's Cookie) 11.6
flaked (Baker's Angel Flake) 11.0
shredded (Baker's Premium Shred) 12.3
shredded (Baker's Southern Style) 10.0
toasted (Baker's Crunchies) 9.7
chocolate flavor (Durkee) 11.8
lemon flavor (Durkee) 11.6
orange flavor (Durkee) 11.6
peppermint flavor (Durkee) 11.6
ginger, crystallized (Borden) 24.2
ginger, preserved (Borden) 22.0

CAKE FROSTINGS, one can or packaged mix*

See also "Dessert Cake Mixes"

	GRAMS
butterscotch, ready to serve (Betty Crocker), 16½-oz. can	333.1
cherry, creamy, mix, prepared** (Betty Crocker), 14.3-oz. pkg.	366.4
chocolate, ready to serve (Betty Crocker), 16½-oz. can	299.8
chocolate, milk, ready to serve (Betty Crocker), 16½-oz. can	326.8
chocolate, fluffy, mix, prepared** (Betty Crocker), 7.2-oz. pkg.	164.2
chocolate fudge, mix, prepared** (Betty Crocker), 15.4-oz. pkg.	376.1
fudge, dark Dutch, ready to serve (Betty Crocker), 16½-oz. can	295.9
lemon, Sunkist, ready to serve (Betty Crocker), 16½-oz. can	336.0
vanilla, ready to serve (Betty Crocker), 16½-oz. can	335.0
white, fluffy, mix, prepared** (Betty Crocker), 7.2-oz. pkg.	195.8

* *The canned and prepared mixes listed here provide enough frosting to ice an eight- or nine-inch layer cake or an oblong cake, 13" x 9" x 2". To determine the carbohydrate content of one slice of cake prepared from a mix and iced with a canned or*

packaged frosting, simply combine the grams in the whole cake with the grams in the frosting, and divide the total by the number of uniform-size slices you've cut. For example, if a "finished" cake contains 654 grams (358 grams of cake, plus 296 grams of frosting) and is cut into twelve uniform-size slices, each slice has 54.5 grams of carbohydrate

** *According to package directions*

CHAPTER 22

CANDY
AND CHEWING GUM

CANDY, one ounce

See "How to Use This Book" (pages 19-23), to learn how to determine the number of ounces—and, therefore, the number of carbohydrate grams—in any specific candy bar, roll, etc.

	GRAMS
(Black Cow Sucker)	20.5
bridge mix (Nabisco)	19.5
see also individual listings, e.g., "nuts, chocolate coated"	
(Butterfinger)	21.0
butterscotch (Nestlé Morsels)	17.0
butterscotch drops, see "hard candy," page 199	
caramel:	
(Whirligigs)	23.2
chocolate (Kraft)	21.3
chocolate (Sugar Daddy Junior)	23.9
coconut (Kraft)	20.5
vanilla (Kraft)	21.4
vanilla (Sugar Babies)	24.7
vanilla (Sugar Daddy Giant)	24.9
vanilla (Sugar Daddy Junior)	24.9
vanilla (Sugar Daddy Nuggets)	24.9

caramel, continued

vanilla (Sugar Daddy Sucker) 24.7
vanilla (Sugar Mama) 22.1
walnut, w/nut slivers (Walnettos) 21.0

caramel, chocolate covered:

vanilla (Kraft) 19.2
vanilla (Kraft Caramelettes) 19.5
vanilla (Milk Duds) 20.5
vanilla (Pom Poms) 20.3
w/nuts, see "nuts and caramel, chocolate covered," page 201

cherries:

dark chocolate covered (Nabisco) 21.9
dark chocolate covered (Welch's) 21.9
milk chocolate covered (Nabisco) 22.1
milk chocolate covered (Welch's) 22.1

chocolate, solid:

bittersweet, see "semisweet," below
milk (Ghirardelli—bars) 16.7
milk (Ghirardelli—block) 16.4
milk (Hershey—bar) 15.9
milk (Hershey—block) 17.8
milk (Hershey Chips) 15.9
milk (Hershey Kisses) 15.9
milk (Kraft Stars) 17.2
milk (Lindt) 15.3
milk (Nabisco Stars) 15.8
milk (Nestlé) 13.1
milk (Nestlé Morsels) 17.3
mint (Ghirardelli) 16.6
mint (Nestlé Morsels) 18.1
semisweet (Eagle) 16.7
semisweet (Ghirardelli Chips) 17.8
semisweet (Hershey Chips) 17.2
semisweet (Hershey Mini-Chips) 17.2
semisweet (Hershey Special Dark) 17.0
semisweet (Lindt Excellence) 13.7
semisweet (Nestlé) 17.3

chocolate, continued

    semisweet (Nestlé Morsels) 18.1
    semisweet, w/vanilla (Lindt) 14.0
    sweet (Hershey Sprigs) 18.3
chocolate, candy coated (Hershey-Ets) 21.0
chocolate, candy coated (M & M's) 18.0
chocolate, with fruit and/or nuts:
    w/almonds (Gala Bar—milk chocolate) 13.9
    w/almonds (Gala Bar—sweet milk chocolate) 14.6
    w/almonds (Ghirardelli) 15.6
    w/almonds (Hershey) 13.8
    w/almonds (Nestlé) 15.3
    w/fruit and nuts (Nestlé Fruit 'N Nut) 16.5
    w/hazelnuts (Gala Bar) 13.9
    w/peanuts (Mr. Goodbar) 12.5
    w/raisins (Ghirardelli) 16.9
chocolate, with crisps and/or bits:
    w/crisped rice (Ghirardelli) 16.7
    w/crisped rice (Krackel) 15.0
    w/crisped rice (Nestlé Crunch) 17.8
    w/malted milk bits (Nabisco Crunch) 16.3
    w/malted milk bits and almond chips
      (Peter Paul Almond Cluster) 16.2
coconut, chocolate covered:
    (Hershey Coconut Cream Egg) 20.4
    (Mounds) 16.6
    (Nabisco Squares) 22.8
    (Welch's) 20.4
    w/almonds (Almond Joy) 16.3
crisps, chocolate covered, w/caramel (Caravelle) 19.0
crisps, chocolate covered, w/caramel ($100,000) 18.9
fudge:
    (Nabisco Home Style) 20.0
    chocolate or vanilla (Stuckey's) 20.8
    chocolate or vanilla (Walter Johnson) 22.3
    chocolate (Kraft Fudgies) 21.3
    chocolate, w/black walnuts (Stuckey's) 19.0

fudge, continued

chocolate, chocolate covered (Welch's) 19.2

chocolate, w/nuts, chocolate covered (Nabisco) 19.0

fudge roll, with caramel and peanuts:

(Baby Ruth) 21.0

(Oh Henry) 26.5

(Oh Henry—2-lb. size) 29.6

(Power House) 19.5

(Williamson Salted Nut Roll) 15.6

gum drops* 24.8

hard candy:

all flavors (Bonomo Sour Balls) 27.8

all flavors (Jolly Rancher Stix Bars) 25.5

all flavors (Jolly Rancher Stix Kisses) 27.5

all flavors, except mint (Life Savers) 27.1

butterscotch (Nabisco Skimmers) 26.9

mint, all varieties (Life Savers) 26.7

jellied candy:

assorted (Chuckles—20-oz. variety pack) 25.1

assorted (Chuckles Rings) 23.5

assorted (Chuckles Ju-Jubes) 25.0

chocolate covered (Kraft Bridge Mix) 20.2

licorice (Chuckles) 23.6

nougat center (Chuckles) 26.6

orange flavor (Chuckles Slices) 24.1

spearmint flavor (Chuckles Leaves) 23.8

spice flavor (Chuckles Sticks and Drops) 24.4

spice flavor (Chuckles Strings) 24.4

jelly beans* 26.4

licorice (Switzer) 24.0

licorice, red (Switzer Cherry Red) 24.0

licorice jellies, see "jellied candy," above

malted milk balls, chocolate covered (Kraft) 18.1

malted milk balls, chocolate covered (Walter Johnson) 18.9

(Mars) 17.0

marshmallows:

(Campfire) 23.0

marshmallows, continued

    (Chuckles Eggs) 27.0
    (Kraft Jet Puff) 22.8
    (Kraft Jet Puff Miniatures) 23.0
    chocolate (Kraft Jet Puff) 21.7
    coconut, toasted (Kraft Jet Puff) 20.4
    flavored (Kraft Jet Puff) 22.8
    flavored (Kraft Jet Puff Miniatures) 23.0
(Milky Way) 19.0
mints, after dinner:
    assorted (Merri-Mints) 28.2
    butter (Kraft) 25.9
    butter (Richardson) 27.0
    butter, colored (Kraft Party) 25.9
    butter, colored (Richardson Pastel) 28.0
    w/jelly center (Richardson) 26.0
    midget (Richardson) 27.0
    striped (Richardson) 28.0
mints, chocolate covered:
    (Junior) 23.0
    (Kraft Minettes Bridge Mix) 19.7
    (Nabisco Mint Wafers) 15.8
    (Nabisco Peppermint Patties) 24.0
    (Nabisco Thin) 22.8
    (Richardson Peppermint Patties) 27.0
(Nabisco Coco-Mello) 19.8
(Nabisco Crispy Clusters) 24.5
nut brittle:
    cashew (Planters Cashew Crunch) 14.4
    peanut (Planters Peanut Block) 14.0
    peanut (Stuckey's) 20.9
    peanut-coconut (Kraft) 21.7
(Nutty Crunch) 19.0
nuts, chocolate covered:
    almonds (Kraft) 11.4
    almonds (Kraft Bridge Mix) 11.5

nuts, chocolate covered, continued
 Brazil (Kraft) 9.0
 peanuts (Kraft) 12.1
 peanuts (Kraft Bridge Mix) 10.0
 peanuts (Nabisco) 11.1
 peanuts, candy coated (Hershey) 17.9
 peanuts, candy coated (M & M's) 16.0
nuts and caramel, chocolate covered:
 almond cluster (Kraft) 12.3
 cashew cluster (Kraft) 12.8
 peanut cluster (Kraft) 10.9
 peanut cluster (Royal Cluster) 13.1
 peanut roll, chocolate flavor (Choc-O-Nut) 26.9
 pecan roll (Stuckey's Log) 17.4
 orange jellies, see "jellied candy," page 199
peanut brittle, see "nut brittle," page 200
peanut butter, chocolate covered (Reese's Peanut Butter Cups) ...15.4
peanut butter, chocolate covered (Reese's Peanut Butter Eggs) ...12.4
peanut crunch (Kraft Bridge Mix) 18.7
popcorn, caramel coated w/nuts (Cracker Jack) 27.3
praline, coconut (Stuckey's) 21.1
praline, maple (Stuckey's) 21.1
raisins, chocolate covered (Kraft) 18.8
raisins, chocolate covered (Nabisco) 20.0
(Rally Bar) 15.5
(Slo-Poke Sucker) 21.0
(Snickers) 16.0
sour balls, see "hard candy," page 199
spearmint leaves, see "jellied candy," page 199
spice drops, see "jellied candy," page 199
taffy:
 all flavors, except chocolate (Bonomo) 25.9
 all flavors, except chocolate (Bonomo Bite Size) 25.9
 chocolate (Bonomo) 23.4
 chocolate (Bonomo Bite Size) 23.6
 molasses (Williamson Kisses) 29.9

Candy, continued

(Three Musketeers) 20.0
toffee:
    almond, chocolate covered (Kraft) 17.9
    chocolate (Kraft) 20.8
    coffee (Kraft) 21.2
    rum butter (Kraft) 21.2
    vanilla (Kraft) 21.2
(Tootsie Roll) 21.5
((Triple Decker) 16.8
(Welch's Frappe) 22.0

* *Data from United States Department of Agriculture*

CHEWING GUM, one piece, except as noted

	GRAMS
(Adams Sour)	2.3
(Beech Nut)	2.3
(Beemans Pepsin)	1.8
(Chiclets)	1.4
(Chiclets—tiny size), 1 package	12.6
(Clorets)	1.3
(Dentyne)	1.3
(Doublemint)	2.3
(Juicy Fruit)	2.4
(Wrigley's Spearmint)	2.2

CHAPTER 23

ICE CREAM AND SIMILAR CONFECTIONS

ICE CREAM & OTHER FROZEN CONFECTIONS,
half cup*, except as noted

	GRAMS
freezing mix, all flavors, prepared** (Junket)	18.2
ice, orange (Sealtest)	32.6
ice bars†:	
chocolate (Popsicle), 3 fl. oz.	23.5
fruit flavors (Kool Pops), 1¼ oz.	8.1
fruit flavors (Popsicle), 3 fl. oz.	16.4
fruit flavors (Sealtest Twin Pops), 3 fl. oz.	17.9
root beer (Popsicle), 3 fl. oz.	16.4
ice cream:	
all flavors, 10.0% fat (Borden)	15.9
all flavors, 10.0% fat (Pet)	13.6
all flavors, 14.0% fat (Lady Borden)	16.9
chocolate, 9.15% fat (Foremost)	17.0
chocolate, 9.8% fat (Sealtest)	17.3
chocolate, 10.0% fat (Carnation)	14.1
chocolate, 10.0% fat (Meadow Gold)	16.5
chocolate, 14.5% fat (Prestige French)	18.0
chocolate chip, 10.0% fat (Carnation)	14.1
strawberry, 8.2% fat (Sealtest)	19.5

ice cream, continued

strawberry, 8.65% fat (Foremost) 15.5

strawberry, 10.0% fat (Carnation) 14.1

vanilla, 10.2% fat (Sealtest) 15.8

vanilla, 10.2% fat (Sealtest Party Slice), 1 slice 15.8

vanilla, 10.35% fat (Foremost) 15.5

vanilla, 12.1% fat (Sealtest) 16.1

vanilla, 16.0% fat (Prestige French) 15.8

vanilla fudge, 8.7% fat (Sealtest Royale) 18.2

ice cream, non-dairy:

all flavors (Meadow Gold) 16.0

chocolate, 10.71% fat (Dutch Pride) 15.5

strawberry, 10.11% fat (Dutch Pride) 15.5

vanilla, 10.65% fat (Dutch Pride) 15.5

ice cream bars†:

chocolate, chocolate coated (Good Humor), 3 fl. oz. 13.6

chocolate, chocolate coated
(Good Humor Whammy-Stix), 1¾ fl. oz. 9.3

chocolate chip, chocolate-malted crunch coated
(Good Humor), 3 fl. oz. 15.1

chocolate chip, chocolate-malted crunch coated
(Good Humor Whammy-Stix), 1¾ fl. oz. 9.5

strawberry, chocolate coated
(Good Humor Whammy-Stix), 1¾ fl. oz. 9.3

strawberry ripple, cake coated
(Good Humor Strawberry Shortcake), 3 fl. oz. 18.3

vanilla, chocolate coated (Good Humor), 3 fl. oz. 13.2

vanilla, chocolate coated
(Good Humor Whammy-Stix), 1¾ fl. oz. 9.1

vanilla, chocolate coated (Sealtest), 2½ fl. oz. 12.1

vanilla, chocolate-toffee coated
(Sealtest Toffee Crunch), 3 fl. oz. 11.9

vanilla, sherbet coated (Creamsicle), 3 fl. oz. 15.6

vanilla, sherbet coated
(Sealtest Orange Creame), 2½ fl. oz. 17.6

vanilla, toasted almond coated (Good Humor), 3 fl. oz. 27.8

vanilla w/chocolate fudge, cake coated
(Good Humor Eclair), 3 fl. oz. 15.6

ice cream cone, vanilla w/chocolate syrup and nuts
(Sealtest Choco-Nut Sundae), 2½ fl. oz. 21.5

ice cream cup, vanilla (Good Humor), 3 fl. oz. 11.6

ice cream sandwich, vanilla w/chocolate wafers
(Sealtest), 3 fl. oz. 26.1

ice milk:

    all flavors, 3.0% fat (Pet) 14.5

    all flavors, 4.0% fat (Pet) 16.8

    buttered almond, 5.3% fat (Light n' Lively) 16.4

    chocolate, 3.1% fat (Light n' Lively) 17.6

    chocolate, 4.4% fat (Foremost Big Dip) 17.0

    orange-pineapple, 2.9% fat (Light n' Lively) 16.7

    peach, 2.6% fat (Light n' Lively) 17.6

    strawberry, 2.7% fat (Light n' Lively) 17.1

    strawberry, 3.7% fat (Foremost Big Dip) 17.0

    vanilla, 4.0% fat (Borden Lite Line) 18.5

    vanilla, 4.0% fat (Meadow Gold) 16.5

    vanilla, 4.2% fat (Foremost Big Dip) 17.0

    vanilla-chocolate-strawberry, 3.0% fat (Light n' Lively) 17.1

    vanilla fudge, 3.3% fat (Light n' Lively) 18.5

ice milk, non-dairy:

    all flavors (Meadow Gold) 17.5

    chocolate, 7.0% fat (Dutch Pride) 13.5

    strawberry, 6.65% fat (Dutch Pride) 14.0

    vanilla, 7.0% fat (Dutch Pride) 14.0

ice milk bars†:

    chocolate, chocolate coated
    (Good Humor Whammy-Stix), 1¾ fl. oz. 10.6

    vanilla, chocolate coated
    (Good Humor Whammy-Stix), 1¾ fl. oz. 10.6

    vanilla, chocolate coated (Sealtest), 2½ fl. oz. 13.6

    vanilla, sherbet coated (Dreamsicle), 2½ fl. oz. 13.0

sherbet:

    fruit flavors (Meadow Gold) 27.5

    fruit flavors, 1.0% fat (Borden) 26.6

    lemon, 1.2% fat (Foremost) 26.0

sherbet, continued

lime, 1.2% fat (Foremost) 26.0
orange (Carnation) 19.7
orange, 1.1% fat (Sealtest) 26.5
orange, 1.2% fat (Foremost) 26.0
pineapple, 1.0% fat (Foremost) 25.0
raspberry, 1.0% fat (Foremost) 25.0
sherbet bars†:
chocolate fudge (Fudgsicle), 2½ fl. oz. 23.4
chocolate fudge (Good Humor), 1¾ fl. oz. 13.4
chocolate fudge (Sealtest), 2½ fl. oz. 18.6
yogurt bar, frozen, see "Yogurt," pages 71, 72

* One quarter pint
** According to package directions
† Note variations in size

ICE CREAM CONES & CUPS, one piece

	GRAMS
cone, plain (Comet)	3.9
cone, assorted colors (Comet)	3.9
cone, rolled sugar (Comet)	10.2
cup, plain (Comet)	4.1
cup, plain (Comet Pilot)	3.9
cup, assorted colors (Comet)	4.1

CHAPTER 24

NUTS, CHIPS, PRETZELS AND RELATED SNACKS

NUTS & SEEDS, SHELLED, one ounce

	GRAMS
almonds:	
barbecued (Blue Diamond)	5.5
blanched, roasted (Funsten)	4.8
blanched, roasted, salted (Blue Diamond)	5.5
blanched, roasted, slivered (Blue Diamond)	5.5
cheese flavor (Blue Diamond)	5.5
dry roasted (Planters)	5.5
dry toasted (Franklin)	5.3
French fried (Blue Diamond)	5.5
onion-garlic flavor (Blue Diamond)	5.5
smoke flavor (Blue Diamond)	5.5
Brazil nuts*	3.1
butternuts*	2.4
cashews:	
dry roasted (Planters)	7.9
dry roasted (Skippy)	8.4
dry toasted (Franklin)	7.7
oil roasted (Planters)	7.8
oil roasted (Skippy)	8.0
chestnuts, fresh*	11.9

Nuts & Seeds, Shelled, *continued*
chestnuts, dried* 22.3
coconut, see "Fruits, Fresh," page 25
filberts, dry toasted (Franklin) 4.5
hickory nuts* 3.6
litchi nuts* 20.1
macadamia nuts* 4.5
mixed nuts:
  w/peanuts, dry roasted (Planters) 6.2
  w/peanuts, dry roasted (Skippy) 6.3
  w/peanuts, dry toasted (Franklin Party Mix) 6.2
  wo/peanuts, dry toasted (Franklin Club Mix) 6.6
  w/peanuts, oil roasted (Planters) 6.2
  w/peanuts, oil roasted (Skippy) 5.9
  wo/peanuts, oil roasted (Planters) 6.0
peanut crisps (Planters) 6.2
peanuts:
  dry roasted (Lay's) 5.2
  dry roasted (Planters) 5.4
  dry roasted (Skippy) 5.4
  w/jackets, dry toasted (Franklin) 6.1
  wo/jackets, dry toasted (Franklin) 6.0
  oil roasted (Nab) 5.3
  oil roasted (Planters) 5.0
  oil roasted (Skippy) 5.2
  Spanish, dry roasted (Planters) 3.4
  Spanish, oil roasted (Planters) 3.4
pecans, raw (Funsten) 3.5
pecans, dry roasted (Planters) 3.5
pepitas, dry toasted (Franklin) 4.1
pistachios, dry toasted (Franklin) 5.1
pumpkin seeds*, dry, hulled 4.3
sesame seeds*, dry, hulled 5.0
squash seeds*, dry, hulled 4.3
sunflower seeds*, dry, hulled 5.6
walnuts, black (Funsten) 3.7

Nuts & Seeds, Shelled, continued

walnuts, English (Diamond) 3.7

walnuts, English (Funsten) 3.9

* *Data from United States Department of Agriculture*

POPCORN & PRETZELS

GRAMS

popcorn:

    plain (all brands), 1 cup, popped 10.3

    butter flavor (Jiffy Pop), 1 cup*, popped 5.9

    butter flavor, ready to eat (Old London), 1 cup 9.9

    butter flavor, ready to eat (Wise), 1 cup* 5.8

    caramel coated, see "Candy," page 201

    cheese flavor, ready to eat (Old London), 1 cup 10.8

    cheese flavor, ready to eat (Wise), 1 cup* 5.8

    seasoned, ready to eat (Old London), 1 cup 9.9

pretzels, one piece**:

    bite-size (Bachman B's) 1.4

    bite-size (Bachman Nutzels) 1.1

    bite-size (Old London Pretz-l Nuggets) 7

    bite-size (Pepperidge Farm Goldfish) 5

    logs (Bachman) 3.1

    logs (Keebler) 3.3

    3-ring (Bachman Beers) 9.8

    3-ring (Bachman Medium) 3.5

    3-ring (Bachman Teeny) 1.9

    3-ring (Bachman Thin) 3.2

    3-ring (Mister Salty) 2.3

    3-ring (Mister Salty Dutch) 11.1

    3-ring (Mister Salty Pretzelettes) 1.3

    3-ring (Mister Salty Veri-Thin) 4.1

    3-ring (Nab Pretzelettes) 1.7

pretzels, one piece, continued

3-ring (Old London Pretz-Is) 1.9
3-ring (Sunshine Extra Thin) 4.0
rods (Bachman) 8.8
sticks (Bachman Stix) 4
sticks (Keebler Stix) 4
sticks (Mister Salty Veri-Thin) 2
sticks (Nab Veri-Thin) 2

* *Packed very loosely*
** *Differences in the size and shape of various brands of pretzels make it almost impossible to compare their carbohydrate content by the piece. For convenience, pretzels are listed here by the piece; however, for accuracy, bear in mind that most brands of pretzels contain approximately 21 to 22 grams of carbohydrate per ounce*

CHIPS, CRISPS, PUFFS, RINDS & STICKS, one ounce

GRAMS

chips, corn:
(Fritos) 15.1
(Nabisco Corn Diggers) 17.1
(Old London) 14.6
(Old London Dipsy Doodles) 14.6
(Wise) 14.8
(Wonder) 14.8
barbecue flavor (Wise) 15.2
chips, corn, popped (Frito-Lay Intermission) 15.9
chips, dip (Nabisco Shapies) 13.0
chips, dip (Nabisco Sip 'N Chips) 17.1
chips, potato:
(Frito-Lay Ruffles) 13.8
(Lay's) 13.8
(Nabisco Chipsters) 19.0
(Wise) 14.6
(Wise Ridgies) 14.6

chips, potato, continued

(Wonder) 13.9
barbecue flavor (Lay's) 13.8
barbecue flavor (Wise) 15.9
barbecue flavor (Wonder) 13.9
onion-garlic flavor (Wise) 15.9

chips, taco (Old London) 16.3
chips, taco-tortilla (Wonder) 17.2
chips, tortilla (Frito-Lay Doritos) 18.1
chips, tortilla (Old London) 16.3
chips, tortilla (Wonder) 17.2

crisps:

(Frito-Lay Fandangos) 15.1
(Frito-Lay Munchos) 15.6
(General Mills Barbecue Vittles) 18.2
(General Mills Bows) 15.0
(General Mills Bugles) 15.0
(General Mills Daisy*s) 17.6
(General Mills French Fried Potato Crisps) 15.0
(General Mills Pizza Spins) 16.0
(General Mills Whistles) 16.0
(Nabisco Doo Dads) 17.4
(Nabisco Korkers) 16.1
(Snow's Clam Crisps) 14.9
(Snow's Onion Crisps) 15.9
(Wise Pizza Wheels) 15.8
(Wonder Corn Capers) 15.4

puffs, cheese flavor or coated:

(Frito-Lay Chee●tos) 15.0
(Jax Cheese Twists) 16.9
(Nabisco Flings) 10.7
(Nabisco Swiss 'N Ham Flavor Flings) 12.9
(Old London Cheez Doodles) 17.3
(Wise Cheese Pixies) 14.6
(Wonder Cheese Twists) 14.7

rinds, fried:

bacon (Wise Bakon Delites) 0

rinds, fried, continued

bacon (Wonder) 0

bacon, barbecue flavor (Wise Bakon Delites) 0

pork (Frito-Lay Baken•ets) ....,...................0

rings, onion flavor:

(Frito-Lay Funyons) 17.8

(Old London) 21.2

(Wise) 22.1

(Wonder) 19.5

shells (Nabisco Shapies) 14.1

sticks, potato (O & C) 14.2

sticks, potato (Wise Julienne) 14.8

sticks, sesame-cheese flavor (Twigs) 16.4

CHAPTER 25

MILK, CREAM
AND SIMILAR PRODUCTS

MILK, eight-ounce glass, except as noted

See also "Milk Beverages, Flavored"

	GRAMS
buttermilk:	
0.1% fat (Borden)	9.8
0.1% fat (Pet)	11.7
0.1% fat (Sealtest Skimmilk)	9.3
0.5% fat (Borden)	9.5
0.5% fat (Meadow Gold)	12.0
0.8% fat (Golden Nugget)	10.0
0.8% fat (Light n' Lively)	10.5
1.0% fat (Borden)	9.5
1.5% fat (Borden)	9.5
1.5% fat (Foremost)	11.2
2.0% fat (Borden)	9.5
2.0% fat (Sealtest Lowfat)	9.3
2.2% fat (Borden)	12.5
3.5% fat (Borden)	9.3
3.5% fat (Sealtest Bulgarian)	11.0
condensed, sweetened, canned:	
(Borden Dime Brand), ¼ cup	42.0
(Borden Eagle Brand), ¼ cup	41.0

condensed, sweetened, canned, continued

(Borden Magnolia Brand), ¼ cup 42.0
(Sealtest), ¼ cup 43.6
dry, reconstituted*:
nonfat (Borden) 11.6
nonfat (Carnation) 11.6
nonfat (Foremost Milkman) 12.2
nonfat (Pet Instant) 12.0
nonfat (Sannalac) 11.0
nonfat (Sealtest) 11.6
whole (Sealtest) 8.5
evaporated, canned:
(Borden Brands), ½ cup 12.2
(Carnation), ½ cup 12.3
(Golden Key), ½ cup 12.0
(Pet), ½ cup 12.0
(Sego), ½ cup 12.0
(Sealtest), ½ cup 12.0
skim (Pet 99), ½ cup 13.0
frozen concentrate (Sealtest), 2 oz. 7.6
half and half, see "Cream," below
skim or nonfat:
0.1% fat (Borden) 11.2
0.1% fat (Pet) 11.7
0.1% fat (Profile Nonfat) 13.0
0.1% fat (Sealtest) 11.3
0.4% fat (Sealtest Diet Skim) 13.8
0.5% fat (Meadow Gold) 13.0
0.5% fat (Profile Skim) 13.0
fortified, 0.1% fat (Borden) 11.2
fortified, 0.1% fat (Borden Vitamin A & D) 11.2
fortified, 0.1% fat (Gail Borden) 11.2
fortified, 1.0% fat (Borden Lite Line) 14.4
fortified, 1.0% fat (Light n' Lively) 13.6
fortified, 1.5% fat (Borden) 15.2
fortified, 1.75% fat (Borden Lifeline) 14.0

skim or nonfat milk, continued

fortified, 2.0% fat (Borden Hi-Protein) 13.9
fortified, 2.0% fat (So-Lo) 13.0
fortified, 2.0% fat (Vita-lure) 13.6
fortified, 2.0% fat (Viva) 14.0

whole:

3.25% fat (Sealtest) 10.8
3.3% fat (Foremost) 11.1
3.3% fat (Meadow Gold) 12.0
3.5% fat (Borden) 11.1
3.5% fat (Foremost) 11.1
3.5% fat (Pet) 11.3
3.5% fat (Sealtest) 11.0
3.7% fat (Borden Cream Line) 11.2
3.7% fat (Pet) 11.3
3.7% fat (Sealtest) 11.1
4.0% fat (Borden) 11.9
fortified, 3.5% fat (Sealtest Multivitamin) 11.0
fortified, 3.7% fat (Gail Borden) 11.2

* *According to package directions*

CREAM, one tablespoon

See also "Creamers, Non-Dairy"

	GRAMS

half and half:

10.5% fat (Borden) 6
10.5% fat (Foremost) 6
10.5% fat (Sealtest) 6
11.5% fat (Borden) 5
12.0% fat (Foremost) 6
12.0% fat (Meadow Gold) 6

half and half, continued

12.0% fat (Pet)	.7
12.0% fat (Sealtest)	.6
heavy, whipping*:	
32.5% fat (Borden)	.5
36.0% fat (Borden)	.5
36.0% fat (Meadow Gold)	.5
36.0% fat (Sealtest)	.5
light, table or coffee:	
16.0% fat (Sealtest)	.6
18.0% fat (Borden)	.6
10.0% fat (Foremost)	.6
18.0% fat (Sealtest)	.6
20.0% fat (Foremost)	.6
medium, 25.0% fat (Sealtest)	.5
medium, whipping*, 30.0% fat (Borden)	.5
medium, whipping*, 30.0% fat (Sealtest)	.5
sour, see "Sour Cream," pages 72-73	
whipped, see "Dessert Toppings," pages 191, 192	

* Unwhipped. Volume is approximately double when whipped

CREAMERS, NON-DAIRY, one tablespoon

	GRAMS
liquid:	
(Coffee Rich)	1.8
(Coffee Twin—frozen)	1.9
(Coffee Twin—liquid)	.9
(Pet Frozen)	1.9
(Meadow Gold Half and Half)	1.2
(Sanna)	2.0
powdered (Coffee-mate)	3.0
powdered (Cremora)	3.0
powdered (Pet)	3.0

EGGNOG*, eight-ounce glass

	GRAMS
canned:	
(Borden Frosted Shake)	41.0
4.7% fat (Borden)	32.5
6.0% fat (Borden)	32.5
8.0% fat (Borden)	32.5
dairy-pack:	
6.0% fat (Foremost)	53.8
6.0% fat (Meadow Gold)	51.0
6.0% fat (Sealtest)	36.0
8.0% fat (Sealtest)	34.6

* *Nonalcoholic*

MILK BEVERAGES, FLAVORED
eight-ounce glass, except as noted

See also "Eggnog" and "Cocoa & Flavored Mixes, Dry"

	GRAMS
cherry-vanilla, canned (Borden Milk Shake)	37.4
cherry-vanilla, mix, prepared* (Foremost Instant Breakfast)	34.2
chocolate:	
canned (Borden Dutch Chocolate Drink)	31.0
canned (Borden Frosted Shake)	40.0
canned (Borden Milk Shake)	37.4
dairy-pack (Borden Dutch Chocolate Milk)	27.1
dairy-pack (Foremost Drink)	18.1
dairy-pack (Foremost Milk)	17.9
dairy-pack (Meadow Gold Drink)	27.0
dairy-pack (Meadow Gold Milk)	27.0

chocolate, continued

dairy-pack (Sealtest Drink—0.5% fat) 26.2
dairy-pack (Sealtest Drink—1% fat) 26.2
dairy-pack (Sealtest Drink—2% fat) 26.1
frozen concentrate, prepared*
(Thick & Frosty Shake—dark chocolate) 41.7
frozen concentrate, prepared*
(Thick & Frosty Shake—light chocolate) 40.4
mix, prepared* (Carnation Instant Breakfast) 34.0
mix, prepared* (Foremost Instant Breakfast—Dutch chocolate) ..34.2
mix, prepared* (Foremost Instant Breakfast—milk chocolate) ...34.2
mix, prepared* (Knox Gelatin Drink), 6-oz. glass 22.1
mix, prepared* (Pet Instant Breakfast Plus) 34.1
mix, prepared* (Pillsbury Instant Breakfast) 36.7
chocolate fudge:
canned (Borden Frosted Shake) 40.0
mix, prepared* (Foremost Instant Breakfast) 34.2
mix, prepared* (Pet Instant Breakfast Plus) 34.1
chocolate malted, mix, prepared* (Pet Instant Breakfast Plus) 34.7
chocolate malted, mix, prepared* (Pillsbury Instant Breakfast) 36.7
coffee, canned (Borden Frosted Shake) 42.0
coffee, canned (Borden Milk Shake) 37.4
coffee, mix, prepared* (Foremost Instant Breakfast) 34.2
mocha, canned (Borden Milk Shake) 37.4
strawberry:
canned (Borden Frosted Shake) 39.0
canned (Borden Milk Shake) 37.4
frozen concentrate, prepared* (Thick & Frosty Shake) 34.2
mix, prepared* (Carnation Instant Breakfast) 35.5
mix, prepared* (Foremost Instant Breakfast) 34.2
mix, prepared* (Pet Instant Breakfast Plus) 35.2
mix, prepared* (Pillsbury Instant Breakfast) 37.9
vanilla:
canned (Borden Frosted Shake) 39.0
canned (Borden Milk Shake) 37.4
frozen concentrate, prepared* (Thick & Frosty Shake) 34.5
mix, prepared* (Carnation Instant Breakfast) 35.4

vanilla, *continued*

mix, prepared* (Foremost Instant Breakfast) 34.2

mix, prepared* (Pet Instant Breakfast Plus) 35.2

mix, prepared* (Pillsbury Instant Breakfast) 35.5

* According to package directions

CHAPTER 26

SOFT DRINKS, COCOA, COFFEE AND TEA

SOFT DRINKS & MIXERS,
eight-ounce glass, except as noted

See also "Fruit & Fruit-Flavored Drinks"
and "Cocktail Mixes, Nonalcoholic"

	GRAMS
birch beer (Canada Dry)	27.0
bitter lemon (Canada Dry)	27.0
bitter lemon (Schweppes)	31.5
blended flavors:	
(Canada Dry Purple Passion)	29.3
(Canada Dry Tahitian Treat)	34.6
(Dr. Pepper)	23.2
(Shasta Tiki)	28.6
cherry:	
(Crush)	32.7
(Fanta)	29.1
black (Shasta)	29.8
wild (Canada Dry)	29.3
citrus (Sprite)	23.2
citrus (Squirt)	23.0
club soda (all brands)	tr.

cola:

(Canada Dry Jamaican) 26.5
(Canada Dry Sport) 26.5
(Coca-Cola) 24.0
(Pepsi-Cola) 26.0
(Royal Crown) 27.4
(Shasta) 26.0
cherry flavored (Shasta) 26.0
collins mixer (Canada Dry) 22.1
cream soda (Canada Dry) 31.9
cream soda (Fanta) 32.3
cream soda (Shasta) 28.6
daiquiri mixer (Schweppes), 4-oz. bottle 50.0
ginger ale:

(Canada Dry) 22.1
(Canada Dry Golden) 22.1
(Fanta) 21.2
(Santiba) 20.4
(Schweppes) 21.7
ginger beer (Canada Dry) 24.4
ginger beer (Schweppes) 23.5
grape:

(Canada Dry Concord) 31.9
(Crush) 34.2
(Fanta) 31.8
(Shasta) 29.8
grapefruit (Fanta) 28.8
grapefruit (Shasta Swing) 28.6
grapefruit (Wink) 30.7
half and half mixer (Canada Dry) 28.3
lemon sour mixer (Canada Dry) 24.4
lemon-lime (Canada Dry) 31.2
lemon-lime (Seven-Up) 24.0
lemon-lime rickey (Canada Dry) 24.4

Soft Drinks & Mixers, continued

orange:

    (Canada Dry Sunshine) 31.9

    (Crush) 31.6

    (Fanta) 31.8

    (Shasta) 32.5

orange-pineapple (Canada Dry Cactus Cooler) 29.3

quinine water (Fanta) 20.4

quinine water (Santiba) 20.4

quinine water (Shasta) 19.2

raspberry, wild (Shasta) 29.8

root beer:

    (Canada Dry Rooti) 26.8

    (Dad's) 26.3

    (Fanta) 30.7

    (Hires) 23.7

    (Shasta) 28.6

screwdriver mixer (Canada Dry) 26.0

sour mixer (Canada Dry) 24.4

strawberry:

    (Canada Dry) 29.3

    (Crush) 32.8

    (Fanta) 30.2

    (Shasta) 27.4

tonic water (Canada Dry) 23.6

tonic water (Schweppes) 22.0

whiskey sour mixer (Canada Dry) 24.4

whiskey sour mixer (Schweppes), 4-oz. bottle 51.2

COCOA & FLAVORED MIXES, DRY, one ounce*

See also "Milk Beverages, Flavored"

	GRAMS
cocoa (EverReady)	22.8
cocoa (Hershey Hot Mix)	21.6

Cocoa & Flavored Mixes, Dry, continued

cocoa, unswt. (Hershey) 13.2
chocolate flavored mixes:
   (Borden Dutch) 25.0
   (Flick Instant) 25.5
   (Hershey Instant) 25.3
   (Nestlé Quik) 25.5
chocolate fudge (Nestlé Quik) 25.5
malted, chocolate flavor (Borden Instant Mix) 23.9
malted, chocolate flavor (Sealtest) 22.8
malted, natural flavor (Borden Instant Mix) 20.1
strawberry (Nestlé Quik) 28.2
vanilla (Nestlé Quik) 27.8

* *Approximately three heaping teaspoonfuls*

COFFEE & TEA, six-ounce cup, except as noted

GRAMS

coffee:
   ground-roasted, prepared* (Chase & Sanborn) 1
   ground-roasted, prepared* (Max-Pax) 5
   ground-roasted, prepared* (Maxwell House) 4
   ground-roasted, prepared* (Sanka) 4
   ground-roasted, prepared* (Yuban) 4
   freeze-dried, prepared* (Maxim) 9
   freeze-dried, prepared* (Sanka) 8
   freeze-dried, prepared* (Taster's Choice) 6
   instant, prepared* (Chase & Sanborn) 1
   instant, prepared* (Decaf) 6
   instant, prepared* (Kava) 6
   instant, prepared* (Maxwell House) 9
   instant, prepared* (Nescafé) 7
   instant, prepared* (Sanka) 9
   instant, prepared* (Siesta) 1

coffee, continued

    instant, prepared* (Yuban) 9

tea:

    bags, prepared* (Crosse & Blackwell) 4

    bags and loose, prepared* (Lipton) ....tr.

    bags, prepared* (Tender Leaf) ....tr.

    instant, prepared* (Lipton) ....tr.

    instant, prepared* (Nestea) 1

    instant, prepared* (Tender Leaf) ....tr.

    instant, lemon flavored, prepared* (Lipton) 7

tea, iced, presweetened, eight-ounce glass:

    canned, ready to serve (Lipton) 34.6

    instant, prepared* (Nestea) 15.1

    instant, prepared* (Salada) 17.6

    instant, prepared* (Tender Leaf) 14.2

    instant, lemon flavored, prepared* (Lipton) 25.5

    instant, lemon flavored, prepared* (Salada) 14.0

    instant, mint flavored, prepared* (Salada) 18.4

* *According to package directions*

CHAPTER 27

SPIRITS, WINES, BEER AND RELATED DRINKS

DISTILLED SPIRITS, one fluid ounce

Applejack, bourbon, brandy, gin, rum, tequila, vodka and every kind of blended and bonded whiskey are known as "distilled spirits" or, if you prefer, straight liquor. As you can see from the single listing that follows, all *unflavored* distilled spirits contain only a trace of carbohydrate per ounce, no matter what brand they are or what their proof (alcoholic content). Most low-carbohydrate plans allow the dieter to drink straight liquor and dry wine "in moderation"; however, there are two notable exceptions: Dr. Stillman's High-Fat, High-Protein Diet and Dr. Atkins' Diet Revolution. On the former plan, no alcohol at all is permitted; on the latter plan, alcohol is forbidden during the first week of dieting and limited strictly thereafter. If you are following, or if you intend to follow, a specific low-gram diet, check the rules carefully; find out if, when, and how much alcohol is allowed.

GRAMS

all distilled spirits, any proof* ....tr.

* *Data from United States Department of Agriculture*

COCKTAILS, BOTTLED, ALCOHOLIC, three fluid ounces

See also "Cocktail Mixes, Nonalcoholic"
and "Distilled Spirits"

	GRAMS
daiquiri (Calvert)	9.5
daiquiri (Hiram Walker)	12.0
mai tai (Lemon Hart)	15.6
Manhattan (Calvert)	2.0
Manhattan (Hiram Walker)	3.0
Margarita (Calvert)	9.5
martini:	
gin (Calvert)	tr.
gin (Hiram Walker)	tr.
vodka (Calvert)	tr.
vodka (Hiram Walker)	tr.
old fashioned (Hiram Walker)	3.0
Pimm's Cup:	
#1, gin (Julius Wile)	9.9
#2, scotch (Julius Wile)	9.0
#3, brandy (Julius Wile)	9.0
#4, brandy and rum (Julius Wile)	2.7
#5, whiskey (Julius Wile)	3.0
#6, vodka (Julius Wile)	5.4
screwdriver (Old Mr. Boston)	10.5
tequila sour (Calvert)	11.4
whiskey sour (Calvert)	9.5
whiskey sour (Hiram Walker)	12.0

COCKTAIL MIXES, NONALCOHOLIC

See also "Cocktails, Alcoholic" and "Soft Drinks & Mixers"

Bear in mind that the figures that follow pertain to the carbohydrate content of mixes alone, in the measure shown. To

determine how many carbohydrate grams a "finished" drink contains, you must also charge yourself for liquor and any other ingredients added to the mix. If only liquor is added, the extra charge is just a trace of a gram; however, if sugar is added (or if a garnish is eaten), you must calculate the number of grams and include it in the total. Bear in mind too that while most bottled and frozen mixes call for the use of one and one-half ounces of mix, a few recipes call for more mix or less mix. Holland House, for example, suggests using two ounces of bottled mix in a Tom Collins, but only three-quarters of an ounce in a Manhattan. When using a bottled or frozen mix, always check the recipe before doing your calculations; if necessary adjust the figures here accordingly.

	GRAMS
bottled and frozen, one and one-half ounces:	
apricot sour (Holland House)	15.8
black Russian (Holland House)	33.7
blackberry sour (Holland House)	16.5
bloody Mary (Holland House)	3.4
bloody Mary, extra tangy (Holland House)	3.4
cocktail host (Holland House)	16.1
daiquiri (Holland House)	15.8
daiquiri (ReaLemon)	24.0
daiquiri, banana (Holland House)	27.0
gimlet (Holland House)	13.1
mai tai (Holland House)	10.5
Manhattan (Holland House)	9.8
Margarita (Holland House)	13.1
martini, dry (Holland House)	3.4
old fashioned (Holland House)	10.9
pina colada (Holland House)	21.8
side car (Holland House)	14.3
Tom Collins (Holland House)	22.1
whiskey sour (Holland House)	16.9
whiskey sour (ReaLemon)	24.0

Cocktail Mixes, Nonalcoholic, continued

dry form, one envelope:

bloody Mary (Bar-Tender's) 5.5
bloody Mary (Holland House) 4.9
daiquiri (Bar-Tender's) 17.0
daiquiri (Holland House) 18.0
Collins (Bar-Tender's) 17.5
Collins, Tom (Holland House) 18.5
gimlet (Holland House) 18.0
mai tai (Bar-Tender's) 17.0
mai tai (Holland House) 18.0
Manhattan (Bar-Tender's) 5.5
Margarita (Bar-Tender's) 17.0
Margarita (Holland House) 18.0
old fashioned (Bar-Tender's) 4.7
screwdriver (Bar-Tender's) 17.5
screwdriver (Holland House) 15.0
vodka sour (Bar-Tender's) 17.0
whiskey sour (Bar-Tender's) 17.0
whiskey sour (Holland House) 18.0

TABLE WINES, four fluid ounces

See also "Aperitif & Dessert Wines"

GRAMS

Beaujolais, see "Burgundy, red," page 229
Bordeaux, French, red (see also "claret," page 230)
château blend (Château La Garde, Chanson Père & Fils) 2.1
château blend (Château Olivier, Chanson Père & Fils) 2.1
district blend, Margaux (B & G) 5
district blend, St. Emilion (B & G) 9
shipper blend (B & G Prince Noir) 5
shipper blend (Chanson Père & Fils Bordeaux Rouge) 2.1

Table Wines, continued

Bordeaux, French, white, dry:

    château blend (Château Olivier, Chanson Père & Fils) 2.1

    district blend, Graves (B & G) 8

    shipper blend (B & G Prince Blanc) 8

Burgundy, red:

    domestic (Gallo) 1.1

    domestic (Gold Seal) 8

    domestic (Italian Swiss Colony Napa-Sonoma-Mendocino) 1.5

    imported, Beaujolais (B & G, St. Louis) 2

    imported, Beaune (Chanson Père & Fils, St. Vincent) 2.1

    imported, Nuits St.-George (B & G) 7

    imported, Pommard (B & G) 5

    imported, Pommard (Chanson Père & Fils, St. Vincent) 2.1

Burgundy, sparkling:

    domestic (Gold Seal) 3.5

    domestic (Italian Swiss Colony) 3.1

    domestic (Lejon) 3.1

    domestic (Taylor) 2.4

    imported (B & G) 2.9

    imported (Chanson Père & Fils) 4.8

Burgundy, white:

    domestic, Chablis (Gallo) 1.2

    domestic, Chablis (Gold Seal) 5

    imported, Chablis (B & G) 2

    imported, Chablis (Chanson Père & Fils, St. Vincent) 2.1

    imported, Pouilly-Fuissé (B & G) 4

    imported, Puligny Montrachet (B & G) 4

Catawba (Gold Seal) 13.0

carousel, pink (Gold Seal) 13.0

carousel, red (Gold Seal) 6.9

carousel, white (Gold Seal) 13.0

Chablis, see "Burgundy, white," above

Champagne:

    domestic, California (Korbel Brut) 9

    domestic, California (Lejon Extra Dry) 2.8

Champagne, continued

    domestic, New York (Gold Seal Brut) 1.9

    domestic, New York (Gold Seal C.F. Brut) 8

    domestic, New York (Taylor Brut) 1.9

    domestic, New York (Taylor Dry Royal Quality) 2.7

    imported (Bollinger Extra Dry) 7.2

    imported (Mumm's Cordon Rouge Brut) 1.9

    imported (Mumm's Extra Dry) 7.5

    imported (Veuve Clicquot Brut) 8

Champagne, pink (Gold Seal Extra Dry) 3.5

Champagne, pink (Lejon Extra Dry) 3.2

Champagne, pink (Taylor) 3.9

Châteauneuf-du-Pape (B & G) 7

Chianti, domestic (Italian Swiss Colony Tipo) 1

Chianti, imported (Brolio Classico) 4

claret (Gold Seal) 5

claret (Italian Swiss Colony Gold Medal) 9

cold duck (Italian Swiss Colony Gold Medal) 5.7

concord (Gold Seal) 13.0

concord (Mogen David) 20.5

Delaware (Gold Seal) 3.5

dinner, red (Taylor Lake Country) 3.9

dinner, white (Gold Seal Fournier Nature) 5

dinner, white (Taylor Lake Country) 2.9

kosher, all dry varieties (Manischewitz) 2.3

kosher, all medium varieties (Manischewitz) 5.7

kosher, all sweet varieties (Manischewitz) 20.5

Liebfraumilch (Anheuser & Fehrs) 1.2

Liebfraumilch (Deinhard) 3.0

Liebfraumilch (Julius Kayser Glockenspiel) 2.4

Moselle:

    Bernkasteler (Deinhard) 5.0

    Graacher Himmelreich (Julius Kayser) 3.3

    Piesporter Riesling (Julius Kayser) 2.3

Nuits St.-George, see "Burgundy, red," page 229

Pommard, see "Burgundy, red," page 229

Pouilly-Fuissé, see "Burgundy, white," page 229

Table Wines, continued

Pouilly-Fumé (B & G) 2
Rhine:
    domestic (Gallo) 1.2
    domestic (Gold Seal) 5
    domestic (Italian Swiss Colony Private Stock) 7
    imported, Niersteiner (Julius Kayser) 1.2
rosé (Gallo) 2.4
rosé (Italian Swiss Colony Gold Medal Grenache) 2.9
rosé (Italian Swiss Colony Napa-Sonoma-Mendocino) 2.9
rosé, sparkling (Nectarose Vin Rosé d'Anjou) 3.4
Sancerre (B & G) 4
Sauterne:
    dry (Gallo) 1.2
    dry (Gold Seal) 6
    dry (Italian Swiss Colony Gold Medal) 9
    dry (Mogen David) 2.0
    semi-dry (Gallo Haut Sauterne) 2.8
    semi-dry (Gold Seal Semi-Soft Sauterne) 3.5
    semi-dry (Taylor) 3.8
Sauternes, see "Aperitif & Dessert Wines," page 232
Zinfandel (Italian Swiss Colony Gold Medal) 9

APERITIF & DESSERT WINES, two fluid ounces

See also "Table Wines"

	GRAMS
Asti Spumante (Gancia)	12.0
(Cherry Kijafa)	10.2
Madeira (Leacock)	6.3
Muscatel:	
(Gallo—14% alcohol)	5.2
(Gallo—20% alcohol)	5.6
(Gold Seal)	6.3

Muscatel, continued

   (Italian Swiss Colony Gold Medal) 6.0
   (Italian Swiss Colony Private Stock) 7.1
   (Taylor) 7.4

Port:

   ruby, domestic (Gallo) 6.3
   ruby, domestic (Gold Seal) 6.3
   ruby, domestic (Italian Swiss Colony Gold Medal) 5.6
   ruby, domestic (Italian Swiss Colony Private Stock) 7.2
   ruby, domestic (Taylor) 7.3
   ruby, imported (Robertson's Black Label) 6.6
   ruby, imported (Sandeman) 6.6
   tawny, domestic (Gallo Old Decanter) 5.6
   tawny, domestic (Italian Swiss Colony Private Stock) 7.0
   tawny, domestic (Taylor) 6.7
   tawny, imported (Robertson's Game Bird) 6.6
   tawny, imported (Sandeman) 6.6

Sauternes (B & G) 5.1
Sauternes (B & G Haut Sauternes) 5.8
Sauternes (Château Voigny, Chanson Père & Fils) 5.0

sherry:

   (Gallo—16% alcohol) 2.2
   (Gallo—20% alcohol) 1.8
   (Gold Seal) 3.1
   (Taylor) 4.7

sherry, cream:

   domestic (Gallo) 5.6
   domestic (Gallo Old Decanter) 8.5
   domestic (Gold Seal) 6.2
   domestic (Italian Swiss Colony) 5.6
   domestic (Taylor) 7.5
   imported (Williams & Humbert Canasta) 3.6

sherry, dry:

   domestic (Gallo) 1.1
   domestic (Gallo Old Decanter) 1.4
   domestic (Gold Seal Cocktail Sherry) 1.1
   domestic (Italian Swiss Colony Gold Medal) 1.1

sherry, dry, continued

domestic (Taylor)	1.9
imported (William & Humbert Dry Sack)	3.0
tokay (Gallo)	5.2
tokay, white (Taylor)	7.6

vermouth, dry:

domestic (Gallo)	1.2
domestic (Lejon Extra Dry)	1.5
domestic (Taylor Extra Dry)	.7
imported (C & P)	2.4
imported (Noilly Prat Extra Dry)	1.1

vermouth, sweet:

domestic (Lejon)	7.6
domestic (Taylor)	6.7
imported (C & P)	9.6
imported (Noilly Prat)	8.0
vermouth, white (Gancia)	5.2

LIQUEURS & OTHER FLAVORED SPIRITS, one fluid ounce

GRAMS

anise-licorice liqueur (DuBouchett Absant)	1.0
anise-licorice liqueur (Leroux Abisante)	1.0
anise-licorice liqueur (Pernod)	1.1

anisette liqueur:

red or white (Bols)	13.9
red or white (DuBouchett)	9.0
red or white (Leroux)	9.9
white (Dolfi)	14.5
white (Garnier)	9.3
white (Old Mr. Boston)	7.5
white (Old Mr. Boston Connoisseur)	8.0

apricot liqueur:

(Bols)	8.9
(Dolfi)	9.8

apricot liqueur, continued

  (DuBouchett) 6.0
  (Leroux) 8.9
(B & B) 5.7
Benai liqueur (DuBouchett) 10.0
Benai and brandy (DuBouchett) 5.0
(Bénédictine) 10.3
blackberry liqueur (Bols) 8.9
blackberry liqueur (Dolfi) 8.1
blackberry liqueur (DuBouchett) 8.0
bourbon, peach flavor (Old Mr. Boston) 8.0
brandy, flavored:
  apricot (Bols) 7.4
  apricot (DuBouchett) 6.0
  apricot (Garnier) 7.1
  apricot (Leroux) 8.6
  apricot (Old Mr. Boston) 8.0
  apricot (Old Mr. Boston Apricot and Brandy) 8.0
  blackberry (Bols) 7.4
  blackberry (DuBouchett) 8.0
  blackberry (Garnier) 7.1
  blackberry (Leroux) 8.3
  blackberry (Leroux Polish) 8.5
  blackberry (Old Mr. Boston) 8.0
  blackberry (Old Mr. Boston Blackberry and Brandy) 8.0
  cherry (Bols) 7.4
  cherry (DuBouchett) 8.0
  cherry (Garnier) 7.1
  cherry, wild (Old Mr. Boston) 8.0
  cherry, wild (old Mr. Boston Wild Cherry and Brandy) 8.0
  coffee (DuBouchett) ....tr.
  coffee (Old Mr. Boston) 1.0
  ginger (DuBouchett) 5.0
  ginger (Garnier) 4.0
  ginger (Leroux) 4.4
  ginger (Leroux Sharp) 4.7
  ginger (Old Mr. Boston) 1.0

brandy, flavored, continued

   ginger (Old Mr. Boston Ginger and Brandy) 8.0
   peach (Bols) 7.4
   peach (DuBouchett) 8.0
   peach (Garnier) 7.1
   peach (Old Mr. Boston) 8.0
   peach (Old Mr. Boston Peach and Brandy) 8.0
(Brighton Punch) 4.0
cherry liqueur:
   (Bols) 8.9
   (Cherry Heering) 10.0
   (Dolfi) 7.8
   (DuBouchett) 8.0
   (Leroux) 7.6
   (Leroux Cherry Karise) 7.6
coffee liqueur (Coffee Southern) 7.0
coffee liqueur (Tia Maria) 10.0
coffee liqueur (Pasha Turkish) 13.3
crème de almond liqueur (DuBouchett) 13.0
crème de almond liqueur (Garnier Crème d'Amande) 15.6
crème de apricot liqueur (Old Mr. Boston) 6.0
crème de banana liqueur (Dolfi Crème de Banane) 13.3
crème de banana liqueur (Garnier Crème de Banane) 11.5
crème de banana liqueur (Old Mr. Boston) 6.0
crème de black cherry liqueur (Old Mr. Boston) 6.0
crème de cacao liqueur:
   brown or white (Bols) 11.8
   brown or white (Dolfi) 14.1
   brown or white (DuBouchett) 16.0
   brown or white (Garnier) 13.1
   brown or white (Old Mr. Boston) 7.0
   brown (Leroux) 14.3
   white (Leroux) 13.3
crème de cassis liqueur:
   (Dolfi) 16.3
   (DuBouchett) 13.0
   (Garnier) 13.5

crème de cassis liqueur, continued

(Leroux) 14.9
crème de menthe liqueur:
  green or white (Bols) 13.0
  green or white (DuBouchett—46 proof) 15.0
  green or white (DuBouchett—60 proof) 13.0
  green or white (Garnier) 15.3
  green or white (Old Mr. Boston) 8.5
  green or white (Old Mr. Boston Connoisseur) 6.0
  gold (DuBouchett) 13.0
  green (Dolfi) 14.0
  green (Leroux) 15.2
  white (Dolfi) 14.2
  white (Leroux) 12.8
crème de noisette liqueur (Dolfi) 11.1
crème de noyaux liqueur (Bols) 13.7
crème de peach liqueur (Old Mr. Boston) 6.0
curaço liqueur:
  blue (Bols) 10.3
  orange (Bols) 8.8
  orange (Dolfi) 9.5
  orange (DuBouchett) 10.0
  orange (Garnier) 12.7
  orange (Leroux) 9.5
(Drambuie) 11.0
gin, flavored:
  lemon (DuBouchett) 1.0
  lemon (Old Mr. Boston) 1.4
  mint (DuBouchett) 3.0
  mint (Old Mr. Boston) 8.0
  orange (DuBouchett) 3.0
  orange (Old Mr. Boston) 1.4
  sloe (Bols) 4.7
  sloe (DuBouchett—48 proof) 8.0
  sloe (DuBouchett—60 proof) 5.0
  sloe (Garnier) 8.5
  sloe (Leroux) 6.0

gin, flavored, continued

   sloe (Old Mr. Boston) 1.4

   sloe (Old Mr. Boston Connoisseur) 2.0

Goldwasser liqueur (Dolfi) 8.5

kirsch liqueur (Garnier) 8

kirsch liqueur (Leroux Kirschwasser) ....tr.

kummel liqueur:

   (DuBouchett—48 proof) 7.0

   (DuBouchett—70 proof) 7.0

   (Garnier) 4.3

   (Leroux) 4.1

   (Old Mr. Boston) 2.0

maraschino liqueur:

   (Dolfi) 11.7

   (DuBouchett) 9.0

   (Garnier) 11.1

   (Leroux) 9.7

peach liqueur:

   (Bols) 8.9

   (Dolfi) 10.6

   (DuBouchett) 8.0

   (Leroux) 8.9

peppermint schnapps:

   (DuBouchett—48 proof) 8.0

   (DuBouchett—60 proof) 9.0

   (Garnier) 8.4

   (Leroux) 9.2

   (Old Mr. Boston) 4.2

   (Old Mr. Boston Connoisseur) 4.5

raspberry liqueur (Dolfi Framberry) 7.3

rock and rum liqueur (DuBouchett) 9.0

rock and rye liqueur:

   (DuBouchett—60 proof) 8.0

   (DuBouchett—70 proof) 8.0

   (Garnier) 6.2

   (Leroux) 8.3

   (Old Mr. Boston) 5.8

rock and rye liqueur, continued

(Old Mr. Boston Connoisseur) 6.0
sloe gin, see "gin, flavored," pages 236-237
sloeberry liqueur (Dolfi Prunelle) 11.0
(Southern Comfort) 3.5
strawberry, wild, liqueur (Dolfi Fraise des Bois) 12.3
tangerine liqueur (Dolfi) 11.3
triple sec liqueur:
  (Bols) 8.8
  (Dolfi) 9.5
  (DuBouchett) 5.0
  (Garnier) 8.5
  (Leroux) 8.9
  (Old Mr. Boston) 10.1
  (Old Mr. Boston Connoisseur) 10.1
vodka, flavored:
  cherry, wild (Old Mr. Boston) 8.0
  grape (Old Mr. Boston) 8.0
  lemon (Old Mr. Boston) 8.0
  lime (Old Mr. Boston) 8.0
  orange (Old Mr. Boston) 8.0
  peppermint (Old Mr. Boston) 5.0

ALE, BEER, & MALT LIQUOR, eight-ounce glass*

	GRAMS
ale (Carling Red Top), 4% alcohol	8.0
beer:	
(Budweiser), 3.6-3.8% alcohol	7.9
(Budweiser), 4.9% alcohol	8.2
(Busch Bavarian), 3.9% alcohol	7.9
(Busch Bavarian), 4.9% alcohol	8.2
(Carling Black Label), 3.6-3.8% alcohol	8.0
(Carlsberg Dark 19-B), 6.5% alcohol	11.2
(Carlsberg Light De Luxe), 4% alcohol	7.2

beer, continued

    (Michelob), 4.9% alcohol 8.5

    (Miller High Life), 3.8% alcohol 8.4

    (Pabst Blue Ribbon), 3.6-3.8% alcohol 8.4

    (Rheingold), 4.6% alcohol 8.8

malt liquor (Champale), 4.7% alcohol 6.2

* *Three-quarters of a "standard" twelve-ounce can or bottle*

WHAT YOU SHOULD WEIGH

WOMEN

height (with shoes—2-in. heels)	small frame	medium frame	large frame
4 ft. 10 in.	92-98	96-107	104-119
4 ft. 11 in.	94-101	98-110	106-122
5 ft. 0 in.	96-104	101-113	109-125
5 ft. 1 in.	99-107	104-116	112-128
5 ft. 2 in.	102-110	107-119	115-131
5 ft. 3 in.	105-113	110-122	118-134 ·
5 ft. 4 in.	108-116	113-126	121-138
5 ft. 5 in.	111-119	116-130	125-142
5 ft. 6 in.	114-123	120-135	129-146
5 ft. 7 in.	118-127	124-139	133-150
5 ft. 8 in.	122-131	128-143	137-154
5 ft. 9 in.	126-135	132-147	141-158
5 ft. 10 in.	130-140	136-151	145-163
5 ft. 11 in.	134-144	140-155	149-168
6 ft. 0 in.	138-148	144-159	153-173

For girls 18-25, subtract 1 pound for each year under 25.

MEN

height (with shoes—1-in. heels)	small frame	medium frame	large frame
5 ft. 2 in.	112-120	118-129	126-141
5 ft. 3 in.	115-123	121-133	129-144
5 ft. 4 in.	118-126	124-136	132-148
5 ft. 5 in.	121-129	127-139	135-152
5 ft. 6 in.	124-133	130-143	138-156
5 ft. 7 in.	128-137	134-147	142-161
5 ft. 8 in.	132-141	138-152	147-166
5 ft. 9 in.	136-145	142-156	151-170
5 ft. 10 in.	140-150	146-160	155-174
5 ft. 11 in.	144-154	150-165	159-179
6 ft. 0 in.	148-158	154-170	164-184
6 ft. 1 in.	152-162	158-175	168-189
6 ft. 2 in.	156-167	162-180	173-194
6 ft. 3 in.	160-171	167-185	178-199
6 ft. 4 in.	164-175	172-190	182-204

Prepared by the Metropolitan Life Insurance Co. from data of the Build and Blood Pressure Study, Society of Actuaries.

INDEX

INDEX

HOW MANY OF THESE DELL BESTSELLERS HAVE YOU READ?